WITHDRAWN

Molecular Genetics of Common Metabolic Disease

Molecular Genetics of Common Metabolic Disease

David J. Galton MD FRCP

Consultant Physician, St Bartholomew's Hospital and
Moorfields Eye Hospital, London

A WILEY MEDICAL PUBLICATION

JOHN WILEY & SONS
NEW YORK

Published 1985
Edward Arnold (Publishers) Ltd.,
41 Bedford Square, London WC1 3DQ

Published in the U.S.A.
by Wiley Medical, a Division of
John Wiley & Sons, Inc., New York

ISBN 0-471-83277-4

Printed in Great Britain

Dedicated to Clare, Sophie and Mitty

Preface

A monograph I wrote on the related topic of 'Errors in Metabolic Regulation' in 1971 contained about ten pages on gene structure and function. The main approach to gene action in humans at that time was a phenotypic study of families for the pattern of inheritance of an abnormal protein or clinical syndrome. This has now changed dramatically and the present monograph is almost all about genes. The change has come about from the isolation and purification of human genes by DNA cloning techniques; of which the globin gene was the first to appear for clinical studies in 1974. There are now some 50 human genes available for study of the fine structure of the human genome or for the study of associated gene polymorphisms. Such an approach when combined with phenotype studies may well provide an insight to the inherited component of such common metabolic diseases as diabetes, hyperlipidaemias and atherosclerosis, that have hitherto defied genetic analysis. It is now possible to study individual genes at the DNA level and assess their contribution to a complex polygenic phenotype. It is also possible to study the structure of regulatory genes that give rise to no definable gene products in the cytoplasm but only affect the activity of other related structural genes. Finally it may be possible to identify genes whose function is as yet unknown but transmit monogenic diseases such as Huntington's chorea or Duchenne Muscular Dystrophy.

It is hoped that the text will primarily interest advanced medical students, clinicians and pathologists interested in diabetes, hyperlipidaemias, atherosclerosis and the other common diseases that have an inherited basis (e.g. hypertension, multiple sclerosis). It is anticipated that the text will not be suitable for research workers in this field since the coverage of topics is designedly at an elementary level and therefore too superficial for their needs; although it may be of help to beginners about to conduct research in this particular area.

This monograph could not have appeared but for the co-operation, assistance, patience and good will of all my colleagues in the Diabetes and Lipid Research Laboratory at St Bartholomew's Hospital, London. Dr. Joseph Stock in particular has been a continuous source of expertise, guidance and loyal support to all in the laboratory. Substantial contributions to the book were made by Laurence Williams and Joseph Stocks (Chapter 3), Simon Wallis (Chapter 4), Alan Rees and Mark Vella (Chapter 6), Graham Hitman and Nigel Jowett (Chapter 7). My colleagues were extremely generous in allowing me to amalgamate and fuse their contributions with the aim of producing a consistent textual style and explaining the material in an elementary manner to Medical Postgraduates assuming no previous background in the subject. The whole monograph has been thoroughly revised and corrected by all of us. Any merit the monograph might possess is entirely due to the efforts of my colleagues; the defects are entirely my own.

David J. Galton
London 1984

Contents

1

Inborn errors of metabolism

The concept of inborn errors of metabolism, as formulated by Archibald Garrod (1857–1936) implies that a single gene defect can give rise to a defective protein to produce disease. His concept applies particularly well to the rare group of metabolic diseases where there are defects in the catalytic activity of enzymes, or defects of receptor or transport function of proteins which are transmitted in families by simple Mendelian inheritance. Diseases such as alkaptonuria, glycogen storage disease and galactosaemia can all arise from single gene mutations affecting key enzymes in metabolic pathways. They are usually transmitted in families by autosomal recessive inheritance; whereas some other single gene defects producing diseases, such as familial hypercholesterolaemia and Huntington's chorea, are transmitted by Mendelian dominant inheritance.

However, the inborn errors of metabolism are individually rare (usual incidence of less than 1:10 000 depending on locality), probably because natural selection is tending to eliminate them from populations. The majority of affected individuals have severe metabolic impairment and fail to reach reproductive age or have reduced fecundity. For example, in phenylketonuria, one of the commoner inborn errors, there is a defect in the activity of phenylalanine hydroxylase in the liver which prevents the conversion of phenylalanine to tyrosine, thereby causing abnormal accumulation of phenyl ketoacids (phenylpyruvic and phenylacetic acids) in the blood and urine. The clinical consequences include failure to thrive, severe mental retardation, epilepsy and eczema. Spread of the mutant gene through populations is therefore reduced, particularly as no known advantage is conferred on individuals with a single dose of the mutant gene (no heterozygous advantage).

Polygenic metabolic disease

However, there is another group of metabolic disorders such as non-insulin dependent diabetes (incidence approximately 1:30), hyperlipidaemia (incidence approximately 1:10 in middle-aged males), and atherosclerosis, all of which occur more frequently in Western populations than any of the classical inborn errors of metabolism. They are responsible for a major health burden in Western societies. Morbidity (diabetic eye disease) and mortality (premature coronary artery disease, cerebrovascular disease, diabetic renal disease) from these three diseases alone far exceed the cumulative effects of all the cancers (Table 1.1). Unlike the inborn errors, the aetiological basis of these three common diseases (non-insulin dependent diabetes, hyperlipidaemia and atherosclerosis) is still incompletely understood. No single mutant protein can be identified as a primary lesion in the majority of cases.

Table 1.1 Representative estimates of mortality of common diseases in England and Wales in 1981

Disease category	Causes of mortality at all ages	
	Male	Female
All causes	289 022	288 868
All neoplasms	66 920	61 771
Chronic bronchitis	11 458	4 153
Ischaemic heart disease	89 104	66 092
Cerebrovascular disease	26 604	43 047
Metabolic disease (mainly diabetes and lipid disorders)	2 547	3 648

Taken from sources: *Review of Registrar General on Deaths by Cause, Sex and Age in England and Wales*, 1981, HMSO; and The Classification of Causes of deaths in the *International Classification of Diseases Injuries and Causes of Death* (revised 1979).

Many previous metabolic studies have suggested that there may be defects in the regulatory properties of rate-determining enzymes or receptor proteins which are otherwise structurally normal. Thus in common forms of primary hypertriglyceridaemia the rate-determining enzyme for the clearance of plasma triglycerides, lipoprotein lipase, is reduced in activity by approximately 50 per cent in some tissues; although the enzyme appears otherwise normal. In some types of non-insulin dependent diabetes the insulin binding activity of cells such as adipocytes may be reduced by about 50 per cent, suggesting a reduced number of cell-surface receptors, although their kinetic properties appear to be normal. Furthermore, although these diseases commonly segregate in families, they do not show the usual patterns of Mendelian inheritance.

Pedigrees can be found in which the disease appears sporadically, or like an autosomal recessive, or like an autosomal dominant. Individuals in the same pedigree can show different phenotypes. Thus some related individuals may have hypercholesterolaemia, others hypertriglyceridaemia, and others a combined hyperlipidaemia, with impaired glucose tolerance variably represented (see Fig. 1.1). For these reasons, polygenic or multifactorial inheritance has been postulated, where two or more genes are inherited which confer a liability to develop the disease when the appropriate environmental factors are encountered. A model for this type of inheritance is shown in Fig. 1.2. The two inner circles contain individuals with a genetic predisposition to develop diabetes, hyperlipidaemia, or both (where the circles overlap); and the outer circle is the general population with a normal genotype. The shaded sectors represent environmental factors (for example excess dietary intake of carbohydrate or fat), which when they overlap with the genetically predisposed individuals will cause appearance of the disease (diabetes and/or hyperlipidaemia).

Such a model can explain several puzzling features of these common metabolic diseases. Firstly, their relative frequency in populations may

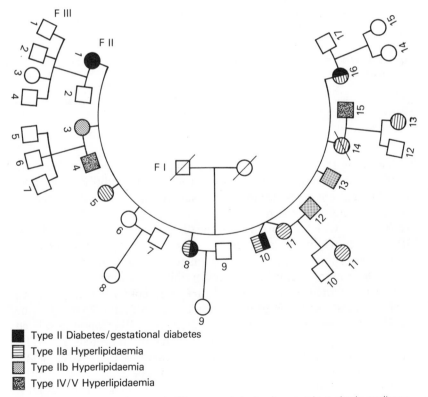

■ Type II Diabetes/gestational diabetes
▤ Type IIa Hyperlipidaemia
▦ Type IIb Hyperlipidaemia
▨ Type IV/V Hyperlipidaemia

Fig. 1.1 Segregation of several different metabolic diseases in a single pedigree.

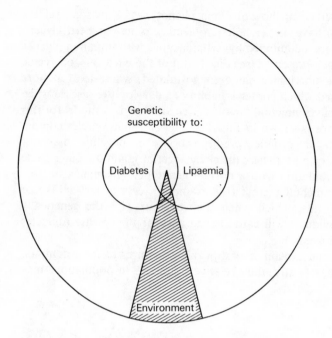

Fig. 1.2 A model of polygenic inheritance. The outer circle represents the normal population; the two inner circles individuals who are genetically predisposed to develop diabetes and/or lipaemia. The hatched sector represents environmental factors (e.g. dietary intake of carbohydrate or fat), which when overlapping with genetically predisposed individuals leads to disease.

be due to the fact that the genes conferring susceptibility may be at no selective disadvantage under most environmental conditions, and may indeed be quite widespread in healthy subgroups as part of the genetic polymorphisms underlying population diversity (see Chapter 5). Secondly, the variable expression of the disease in families may be due to differences in relative duration and severity of the environmental factors to which individuals are exposed or to the requirements of more than one genetic determinant. Thirdly, the 'susceptibility' genes may not code for a particular protein (enzyme or cell-surface receptor) but may only be involved in the regulation of expression of such structural genes (i.e. be regulatory genes); hence no mutant protein would be found in related tissues, but only an alteration in the level of a normal protein. Fourthly, they may be much more amenable to therapy by environmental modification (such as dietary restriction), because their genetic component is not deleterious under many environmental conditions, unlike the rare mutations of the inborn errors.

New developments

In the past a direct analysis of a monogenic disease has been made by identification and characterization of the mutant protein in relevant tissues. From the properties of the mutant enzyme or receptor and the pattern of its inheritance in family members, direct inferences can be made of the underlying gene defect. The detection of the mutant protein (present from birth) provides an early means of diagnosis. However, not all monogenic diseases can be identified at an early stage in this way. The mutations underlying Duchenne muscular dystrophy and cystic fibrosis, for example, remain to be discovered, so early diagnosis of both diseases rely on the first presentation of the clinical features of each disease.

In the case of the common metabolic diseases it is not even expected that a mutant protein forms the primary lesion of the disease. Early diagnosis of non-insulin dependent diabetes or the hyperlipidaemias is currently established by measurement of the appropriate metabolite (glucose or lipids) accumulating in the blood. If above certain arbitrarily defined limits, usually defined by the upper limit of distribution of the metabolite in a healthy population from the same geographical locality (Fig. 1.3) the diagnosis is established. Although the genetic predisposition to the disease is present from birth, the age of onset of the disease can be extremely variable, spanning childhood to old age. The problem in the early stages of the disease is knowing whether an individual in the right hand part of the curve of Fig. 1.3 (shaded area) falls within the normal distribution of the population, or is an affected

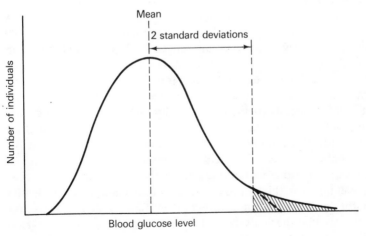

Fig. 1.3 Frequency distribution of blood glucose in a population. The distribution curve is skewed to the right. Individuals in this tail may either be at the upper limit of a normal distribution or have diabetes mellitus.

individual with the disease, particularly when the distribution is skewed to the right. Loading or stress tests, such as the glucose tolerance, fat-meal or intralipid tests sometimes help to distinguish between the two. However, a better means to diagnose the early presence of a metabolic disease is to search for the underlying cellular abnormalities (either nuclear or cytoplasmic) that give rise to the abnormal accumulation of metabolites.

There have been some revolutionary new developments in the past five years that enable a direct visualization of human genes, and which may allow a direct assessment of a particular gene's contribution to the disease process. This applies to defects of regulatory genes or promotor or enhancer loci which would never be expected to give rise to a mutant protein in peripheral tissues, but only alter the levels of existing proteins. It also may apply to analysis of the contribution of two or more genes to a disease process. The new developments have been in a series of interrelated biochemical and microbiological techniques that allow:

1. direct isolation of human genes from any cell;

2. transfer of such genes into bacteria such as *E. coli*;

3. cloning of such genes to high yields, and subsequent harvesting for further studies; and

4. rapid sequencing techniques for DNA that permit positive identification of the gene under study by its correspondence with the amino acid sequence of the gene product (if there is one).

All these techniques are described more fully in Chapter 4; but the complexity of the problem can be appreciated from Fig. 1.4. The nucleus of a human cell contains sufficient DNA to code for more than a million genes. Table 1.2 presents the average amounts and distribution of DNA in a typical human nucleus. Probably in any one cell only 10–15 000 genes are functioning to produce messenger RNA (mRNA) for protein synthesis on polyribosomes. The problem is then to identify one out of the many thousand genes in the nucleus; transfer the gene into the DNA of a bacterial plasmid (a plasmid is a piece of bacterial DNA that replicates independently of the bacterial chromosome and often carries genes for antibiotic resistance); grow large amounts of the bacterial plasmid for identification of the inserted human gene; and then use the radiolabelled human gene for identification and study of the genes of patient groups or pedigrees that may be involved in the disease process. Some advantages of this approach, apart from being able to identify contributory genes that do not have an identifiable gene product in the cytoplasm, are that the analysis can be conducted in any cell type even if the gene is not being expressed in that particular cell. For example, the insulin gene is usually expressed only in the β-cell of the islets of the pancreas to make insulin; yet the structure of the insulin gene can be studied in the nuclear DNA of leucocytes, adipocytes, or trophoblast of the foetus. This clearly facilitates a genetic analysis. Also the linkage associations of genes with disease susceptibility can now be studied directly. Previously the effects of genetic linkage could only be analysed in pedigrees, where, for example, the coinheritance of a particular HLA haplotype was seen in affected but not in unaffected siblings. Now the variation in structure of the associated genes can be studied directly in nuclear DNA.

Finally, it has become feasible to undertake a genetic analysis even when the genes responsible for the disease are not known. This involves the use of random lengths of human DNA as genomic probes to see if they coinherit with the disease phenotype in affected pedigrees. If there is

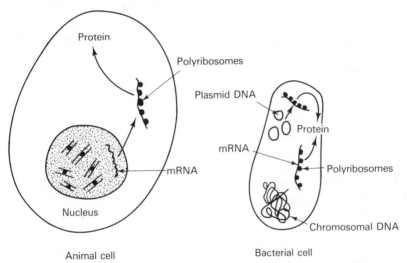

Fig. 1.4 Schematic diagram of a representative animal and bacterial cell (not to scale). Nuclear genes from the animal cell can be transferred into plasmid DNA of the bacterial cell. After many replicative cycles and amplification, the animal DNA can be obtained in large quantities from the plasmids of the bacterial cell.

Table 1.2 The human genome

Size of genome	2.1×10^{12} Daltons
Amount of DNA per haploid genome	1.8 picograms
Number of DNA kilobases per haploid genome	3×10^6 kb
Per cent of unique copy sequences	approx 51%
(slow reassociation component)	
Number of potential genes (if 1 gene $\cong$ 1kb)	approx 1.4×10^6
Number of expressed genes per cell	approx 1×10^4

Taken from sources: Lewin (1980). *Gene expression*, J. Wiley and Sons, New York. Bradbury, Maclean and Mathews (1981). *DNA, Chromatin and Chromosomes*. Blackwell Scientific Publications, Oxford.

a one-to-one correspondence between the appearance of the disease and the presence of an abnormal gene locus (as identified with the genomic probe), then one has found a disease-specific locus that may even be the mutant gene responsible for the disease. Such an approach has been useful in the identification of possible gene loci involved in the production of Duchenne muscular dystrophy (p.116) and Huntington's chorea (p.116).

Genomic probes

One of the most useful products of the recombinant DNA technology for the analysis of genetic disease in man is the gene probe. This is an isolated length of DNA whose nucleotide base sequence is complementary to a base sequence existing in the human genome. This means that the probe will hybridize strongly under proper conditions to its complementary sequence in the genome, rather in the way an antibody will strongly combine with its antigen and provide a means for its localization in tissues.

The technique for localizing genomic sequences in human DNA by hybridization with genomic probes is described in detail using the method of 'Southern blotting' in Chapter 4. Briefly, the procedure is to isolate DNA from human nuclei (leucocytes are a good source for this), cleave the DNA into small fragments by restriction enzymes, separate the DNA fragments by size on gel electrophoresis and hybridize the single-stranded fragments to a radiolabelled genomic probe which is also single-stranded. The probe, under the correct experimental conditions, will bind strongly to its DNA counterpart of the genome and so can be localized by techniques such as autoradiography. The information gained by such methods, is whether one or many gene copies are present in the sample of human DNA and also on what sized fragments the DNA of the gene is contained. This method can be extremely useful in the analysis of groups of patients or pedigrees in which genetic variants are believed to predispose to a disease state. The genetic variants can be identified as different sized fragments by gel electrophoresis and their associations with metabolic disease studied.

Gene probes can be mainly used for four types of related studies in patient groups:

1. For a direct study of the fine structure of the gene suspected to be involved in the disease process; detecting abnormalities of nucleotide sequence; or insertion or deletion of nucleotide sequences in the gene structure.

2. For variation in DNA sequences close to the relevant gene (i.e.

DNA polymorphisms) that may affect gene expressions, or be a genetic 'marker' for adjacent loci involved in the metabolic disease, to allow identification of family members who are at risk.

3. For population and racial distributions of relevant polymorphisms in demographic studies.

4. For study of gene clusters, where genes involved in a particular aspect of metabolism may occur closely together on the same chromosome.

Further reading

Alberts, B., Bray, D., Lewis, J., Raff, M., Roberts, K. and Watson, J.D. (1983). *Molecular Biology of the Cell*. Garland, New York.

Galton, D.J. (1971). *The Human Adipose Cell: A Model for Errors in Metabolic Regulation*. Butterworths, London.
(An early monograph on metabolic disease and disorders of enzyme regulation.)

Garrod, A.E. (1909). *Inborn Errors of Metabolism*. Oxford University Press, Oxford.
(A classical monograph relating metabolic disease to disordered gene function.)

Harris, H. (1980). *Principles of Human Biochemical Genetics*. Elsevier, Holland.
(A comprehensive text on biochemical aspects of modern human genetics.)

Judson, H.F. (1979). *The Eighth Day of Creation: Makers of the Revolution in Biology*. Simon and Schuster, New York.
(An excellent general account of the history of molecular biology.)

Stanbury, J.B., Wyngaarden, J.B., Fredrickson, D.S., Goldstein, J.L. and Brown, M.S. (1983). *The Metabolic Basis of Inherited Disease*, 5th edition. McGraw-Hill Co., New York.

Vogel, F. and Moltusky, A.G. (1980). *Human Genetics: Problems and Approaches*. Springer-Verlag, Berlin.

Wagner, R.P., Judd, B.H., Saunders, B.G. and Richardson, R.H. (1980). *Introduction to Modern Genetics*. John Wiley and Sons, New York.
(One of many excellent introductory texts for undergraduates.)

2

Evolution: significance for metabolic disease

The gene frequencies of animal populations are undergoing continual change with time. Contemporary evolutionary theory proposes this is primarily due to three major influences:

1. the rates of gene mutations in the population;
2. the effect of natural selection (either positive or negative) on the transmission of existing genotypes to succeeding generations; and
3. the effect of genetic drift.

A mutation is a change in the DNA sequence of the genome and occurs at finite but variable rates depending on the locus and animal species. Average values for mutation rates in man are given in Table 2.1. A change in the DNA sequence of a structural gene may have deleterious effects and be gradually eliminated from the population. Many such mutations are the basis for the inborn errors of metabolism. If the mutated gene locus codes for a protein (enzyme, metabolite carrier or receptor) that is just sufficient in activity for its normal function in

Table 2.1 Average values for mutation rates in man for autosomal dominant disorders

Disorder	Mutation rate per gamete	Remarks
Aniridia	0.5×10^{-5}	
Myotonic dystrophy	1.6×10^{-5}	
Huntington's chorea	0.5×10^{-5}	Upper limit
	$0.2 \times 10^{--5}$	More probable limit
Retinoblastoma	1.5×10^{-5}	Probably includes phenocopies
	2.3×10^{-5}	
	0.4×10^{-5}	Corrected for phenocopies
Neurofibromatoma	8×10^{-5}	

Taken from various sources: Cavalli-Sforza, L.L. and Bodmer, W.F. (1971). *The Genetics of Human Populations*. W.H. Freeman and Co., San Francisco.

tissues (that is production of the protein by a single parental locus is insufficient for the body's requirements), then the mutant will be transmitted in families as a dominant disease. If only one parental gene locus is required for normal production of the protein, then the mutation will be recessive, meaning that the heterozygous individual will be healthy (but a carrier) and the disease will only appear when both mutated genes are inherited together, one from each parent.

Although mutation is the structural basis for evolutionary change in populations, many structural gene mutations, i.e. those coding for proteins, are likely to be deleterious because of their association with an abnormally functioning protein. As such, they will be at a selective disadvantage and may decline in frequency in the population to the point of extinction. However, if the gene mutation is recessive there will be a number of subjects carrying a single dose of the mutated gene (heterozygotes) at no or minimal selective disadvantage, so the abnormal gene may persist but only produce disease in offspring when both parents are carriers (heterozygotes). This model of dominant or recessive inheritance of single gene loci is adequate to explain the inheritance of the majority of the rare inborn errors of metabolism. It is not sufficient to account for the inheritance of those common metabolic diseases which occur in more than two per cent of the population. Can their inheritance be explained on the basis of current evolutionary theory?

Genetic diversity

During the millenia of evolutionary time some mutations may be at a selective advantage over the original or 'wild-type' gene and so start to increase in frequency with succeeding generations until it reaches a balance with the original gene. For prevailing environmental conditions the mutation may be neutral with regard to the original gene, so that individuals carrying either genetic variant are equally viable or fertile. The mutated gene may still spread through the population by genetic drift due primarily to random sampling of the parental genotype by succeeding generations of offspring. Large numbers of such mutations can become established in populations and give rise to a considerable degree of genetic diversity within that population. It is of evolutionary advantage for such populations to have a large amount of underlying genetic diversity so as to be able to adapt to changing environmental conditions. Natural selective forces can vary with time and a slightly unfavourable genetic variant may become better fitted for adaptation to the new environmental conditions than the previous genotype. Members of the species with the unusual gene variant will become better adapted to the new selective forces and the species as a whole may survive through them. The underlying genetic diversity of the species may therefore be of considerable evolutionary advantage.

Multiple molecular forms of enzymes

The genetic diversity of man can be observed by several different means. One relevant to metabolism is that enzymic and structural proteins often occur in multiple molecular forms. Within tissues, for example, the enzyme hexokinase, which is responsible for the phosphorylation of glucose after entry into the cell for metabolism by the glycolytic pathway, can occur in four different molecular forms called isoenzymes

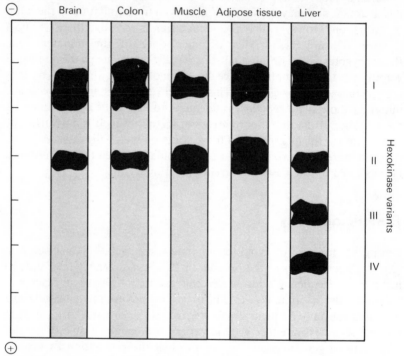

Fig. 2.1 Diagram of multiple forms of hexokinase in human tissues shown by the acrylamide gel electrophoretic pattern of hexokinase types from a 31 000 xg supernatant extracts of homogenates of various human tissues. Gels were stained for hexokinase activity at a substrate concentration of 0.1M glucose. The Type III hexokinase is inhibited at this concentration of glucose and is more clearly evident when the gel is stained at 0.5mM glucose. The bands identifying hexokinase activity result from the reduction of nitro-tetrazolium blue by reduced phenazine methosulphate in a reaction which is coupled to the oxidation of glucose-6-phosphate formed by the hexokinase reaction. The specificity for hexokinase activity was indicated by the lack of colour development in the absence of either ATP or glucose. (Source: Galton, D.J. and Jones, A.E. (1967) *Proceedings of the Society for Experimental Biology and Medicine* **126**, 479.)

(Fig. 2.1). They can be separated by their differences in charge by starch or acrylamide gel electrophoresis. Three of the multiple forms of the enzymes are variously distributed in peripheral tissues and in addition to differences in electrophoretic mobility can be distinguished by differences in stability to heat at 45°C for one hour in the absence of glucose. Many other such examples are known and a list of some of the other enzymes occurring in multiple forms is given in Table 2.2.

Table 2.2 A partial list of enzymes that occur in multiple or single molecular forms

	Enzymes occurring in:		
Enzyme class	Multiple forms	Single form	Total
Oxidoreductases	8	11	19
Transferases	9	11	20
Hydrolases	7	26	33
Lyases	4	3	7
Isomerases	1	2	3
Ligases	—	1	1
	29	54	

Source of data: Harris, H. (1980). *Principles of Human Biochemical Genetics*, Elsevier, Holland.

Such diversity of protein structure can be achieved in two main ways:
1. by variation occurring at a single gene locus, where one allele codes for one protein and the other allele for a slightly different protein structure; or
2. by duplication of genes arising from a single ancestral gene, which have then diverged and now code for slightly different proteins.
Both mechanisms are known to operate. Variation of a single locus can be estimated by the degree of heterozygosity occurring at gene loci.

Extent of heterozygosity
The widespread occurrence of protein polymorphism implies that any individual is likely to be heterozygous at many different gene loci and it is of obvious interest to enquire to what extent heterozygosity occurs. This is the proportion of gene loci in an individual at which there are likely to occur two different alleles each coding for a structurally distinct version of the peptide.

Table 2.3 Extent of enzyme polymorphism in European subjects

Number of loci screened	104
Number of loci showing electrophoretic polymorphism	24
Percentage of polymorphic loci	23
Average heterozygosity (per cent)	6.3

Source: Harris, H. (1980). *Principles of Human Biochemical Genetics*. Elsevier, Holland.

Table 2.3 summarizes the extent of polymorphism occurring in a survey of enzymes analysed by electrophoresis in individuals of European origin. Data on the enzymic products of 104 different gene loci were available and of these loci 24 showed electrophoretic polymorphism. The average heterozygosity is the sum of observed values for heterozygosity at each locus divided by the total number of loci (i.e. 104). This turns out to be 6.3 per cent. This value for heterozygosity is very likely to be an underestimate because:

1. It is derived from electrophoretic data which implies a charge difference in the different molecular forms of the gene product, and some alternative alleles may produce a produce in which a neutral amino acid is substituted and so gives rise to no differences on electrophoresis. Additionally, there are technical difficulties of visualizing variants on electrophoresis.

2. Most surveys are based on enzyme polymorphism, and these may not be representative of other gene-products such as structural or carrier proteins.

3. There is likely to be much more allelic variation at the DNA level that could be influenced by natural selection but does not appear as protein variants.

For example, because of the degeneracy of the genetic code (i.e. two or more nucleotide triplets may code for the same amino acid, see p.29), single base change mutations may alter a codon but still specify the same amino acid. So they produce no change in the structure of the protein, but may affect rates of protein synthesis because of preferred codon usage by the transfer RNAs (tRNAs). Also, DNA variation may occur in the region of intervening sequences (introns) or other non-coding parts of the gene that will not affect the structure of the product, but may affect rates of gene expression and so be subject to the process of natural selection. Some, and perhaps the majority, of allelic variants may of course be neutral with regard to selection forces, but may become advantageous under appropriate environmental conditions or when associated with a different genetic background. Thus neutral mutants have a latent potential for selection. However, the important point to emerge from these studies is the very considerable extent of individual diversity in protein structure that occurs in human populations.

Gene duplication

Hereditary variation by gene duplication, where multiple copies of a slightly different gene occur may be a powerful creative force in evolution (Fig. 2.2). Its extent is less fully established because the means for studying gene structures in mammalian cells have only recently become available. Examples are the duplication of the rat insulin gene,

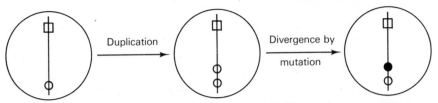

Fig. 2.2 Gene duplication in evolution. The creation of a new gene in a hypothetical haploid cell by duplication, with subsequent divergence by accumulation of mutations during evolutionary time.

where two genes with identical coding sequences, but different intervening sequences, occur on chromosome 11. Both genes are involved in the production of insulin but whether one has selective advantage over the other is not at present known. Other examples of gene duplications are listed in Table 2.4.

Table 2.4 Example of genes which may have arisen by duplication

Gene (organism)	Organization of structural regions	Other comments
Histone (sea urchin)	5 genes arranged in order, no introns	Multiple identical copies of genes repeated in tandem arrays
Ribosomal RNA (fruit fly)	Up to 250 genes, each with one intron	
Ovalbumin (chicken)	3 genes closely homologous and oriented in same direction	Genes separated by large DNA tracts of 6–11kb
Insulin (rat)	2 genes differing by the presence of 1 intron	2 copies close together on chromosome 11
α globin (man)	2 identical genes with introns	2 copies close together on chromosome 16
γ globin (man)	2 genes with at least 1 different codon (γ^G and γ^A globulin)	2 copies close together on chromosome 11
Interferons (man)	At least 8 genes in leucocytes. Only 1 fibroblast gene with no introns	
Immunoglobulins (mouse)	3 unlinked loci: one contains several V_λ and C_λ genes, another contains 100–600 V_K and 1 C_K gene, a third contains 70–400 V_H and 8 C_H genes	

Other examples of multiple genes: collagen, vitellogen, δ-crystallin, actin.

Sources: Lewin, B-(1974). *Gene expression.* John Wiley and Sons, New York.
Bradbury, E.M., Maclean, N., Matthews, H.R. (1981). *DNA, Chromatin and Chromosomes.* Blackwell Scientific Publications, Oxford.

From the evolutionary viewpoint the existence of two copies of the same gene enables one of the copies to accumulate mutations and to eventually emerge as a new gene, while the other copy retains the old function required by the species for survival through the transitional period. Duplications thus enable genes to make evolutionary experiments which have been forbidden before, liberating them from incessant natural selection whose overwhelming effect is to stabilize the genetic status quo. This allows fixation of mutants that are slightly deleterious for contemporary conditions, but which may have other useful effects for adaptation to a new environment. Like ordinary point mutations, gene duplications may be constantly occurring at low frequencies and in the majority of cases may lead to degeneration of one of the duplicated copies into a pseudogene. However, in some cases, the results of gene duplication can be useful and lead to the appearance of multigene families. These represent groups of tandemly repeated genes which are characterized by four properties: multiplicity, close linkage, sequence homology and overlapping phenotype functions. Good examples are the immunoglobulin genes, histone genes and probably the apolipoprotein genes (see Table 2.4).

It is thus seen that there is a considerable degree of allelic and genotypic variation in populations with some variants possibly favouring a slight difference in physiological function of that particular protein. How such genetic diversity is maintained in populations and how natural selection operates to favour the spread of genotypes is not the subject of this volume. Whether such genetic variants could be at a selective disadvantage by association with disease processes is a major topic. The hypothesis that previously evolved genetic variants (either allelic or genotypic) may have had selective advantage in the past, their frequency increasing in the population to more than several per cent, but due to changing environmental conditions are now no longer well-adapted, could account for the genetic basis of the common metabolic diseases. The inherited component of the common metabolic diseases on this hypothesis would be a genetic polymorphism already present at substantial frequencies (greater than one to two per cent) in the population, which is now at a slight selective disadvantage, by association with metabolic disease under particular environmental conditions.

A possible example of such a process may be the polymorphic variants close to the insulin gene that associates with the glucose intolerance; this is described fully in Chapter 7. Briefly, there is a highly polymorphic locus close to the insulin gene on the short arm of chromosome 11. The polymorphism is due to great variation in the insertion of different lengths of simple DNA sequences, ranging from 0–2.5 kb (1kb = 1 000 base pairs). The role of the polymorphic locus is not known. However, individuals who are homozygous for the large insertion sequence occur quite rarely in the population (less than five per cent of healthy subjects); whereas heterozygotes for large and small insertions are relatively common (> 40 per cent). The frequency of the homozygous large allele is increased to > 30 per cent in patients with glucose and lipid intolerance. It is possible that this genotype variant is rare in the general population because of such a disease association and may be declining in frequency by conferring a reduced 'fitness' or viability on such individuals. There are also other disease associations with this polymorphic site considered further in Chapter 7.

Organic evolution requires mutations for the basis of the genetic diversity of populations. Some genetic variants successfully meet environmental challenges in past or present conditions. Others are ill-adapted to prevailing conditions and impose a burden of genetic variants in the population that are deleterious. Some of these may have spread quite widely in the population, possibly due to a previous selective advantage, and are present as polymorphic forms. However, they may now associate with disease and provide the inherited basis of such common disorders as diabetes mellitus, hyperlipidaemia and athero-sclerosis.

Further reading

Bodmer, W.F. and Cavalli-Sforza, L.L. (1976). *Genetics, Evolution and Man*. W.H. Freeman and Co., San Farncisco.
(A very good general account.)
Dobzhansky, T., Ayala, F.J., Stebbins, G.L. and Valentine, J.W. (1977). *Evolution*. W.H. Freeman and Co., San Francisco.
(A modern synthesis of ideas on the premise that nothing in biology makes sense except in the light of evolution.)
Kimura, M. (1983). *Neutral Theory of Evolution*. Cambridge University Press, Cambridge, England.
(A scholarly monograph on the role of neutral evolution.)
Lewontin, R.S. (1983). *Human Diversity*. W.H. Freeman, San Francisco.
(An elementary account of the genetics of human groups.)
Nei, M. and Koehn, R.K. (1983). *Evolution of Genes and Proteins*. Sinauer Association, Massachusetts.
(A series of contributions on DNA polymorphisms and evolution.)
Parkin, D.T. (1979). *An Introduction to Evolutionary Genetics*. Edward Arnold, London.
(Mainly from a zoological viewpoint.)

3
The human genome

All the genetic information of a cell is encoded in long thread-like molecules of DNA. The cellular DNA contains the individual genes arranged along its length and is divided up amongst the 46 separate chromosomes. Genes carry information for the production of all the cellular proteins and can be either arranged individually, separated by large regions of non-coding DNA; or occur closely together in gene clusters or complexes.

Within the body, cellular functions vary widely in different cell types. However, all the cells (with the exception of sperm and egg cells) contain the same genetic information. What accounts for the differences between cell types is the differential expression of the information encoded by the genes. This arises through a complex set of interactions involving the rearrangement, folding and binding to DNA of a variety of DNA-associated proteins during differentiation and throughout adult life.

The human genome was previously considered as a static structure containing a string of basic genetic units joined by covalent chemical bonding; it should now be considered as a much more dynamic structure where the primary structure of DNA is affected by a complex set of interactions with protein to alter the secondary structure and with a variety of insertional elements able to vary the primary structure. In the following sections the structure of DNA will be discussed from the level of the nucleotides to the double helix and its interaction with the DNA-associated proteins; then the structure of genes, their expression and regulation will be briefly considered.

Structure of DNA

The first steps in the analysis of nucleic acids were undertaken some 100 years ago. Initially an unusual nuclear material was found that contained phosphorus, and was called 'nuclein'. Later work identified two forms of nucleic acid: one form associated mainly with the nuclear fraction of the cell called DNA; the other was more labile and found mainly in the cytoplasm, called RNA.

Chemical composition of DNA

The complete hydrolysis of nucleic acids yield compounds containing cyclic ring structures, the purine and pyrimidine bases. The common cyclic bases of DNA are cytosine, guanine, thymine and adenine and are illustrated in Fig. 3.1

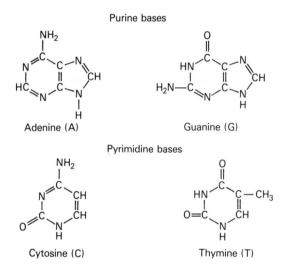

Fig. 3.1 Diagram of the common purine and pyrimidine bases found in DNA.

The involvement of a pentose sugar with nucleic acids was recognized early in the elucidation of DNA structure. It was then shown that ribose was incorporated in the structure of the nucleic acids of the cytoplasm, and deoxyribose in the nuclear associated material. This difference in the sugar residue produces some of the different physical and chemical properties that exist between DNA and RNA. For example, DNA is much more resistant to hydrolysis than RNA; and this becomes important as DNA has to remain stable and intact throughout the cell's life and be exactly replicated for transmission to the next generation. On the other hand, RNA is subject to many cellular control processes and may have a very short half-life within a cell.

Purine or pyrimidine bases are linked to the sugar moiety (either ribose or deoxyribose) to form nucleosides. The latter are then linked to a phosphate group through carbon-5 of the sugar to form nucleotides

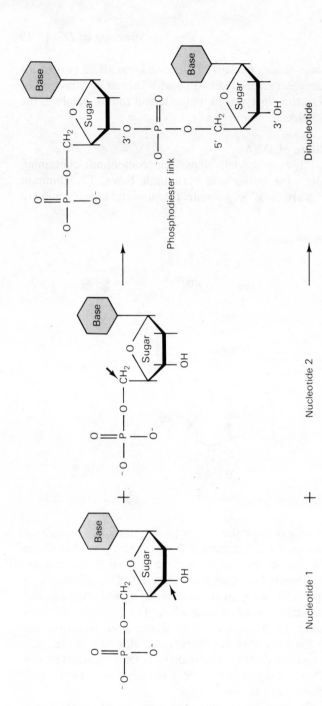

Fig. 3.2 Formation of polynucleotides from nucleotide precursors. Nucleotides are joined together by a phosphodiester linkage to form a nucleic acid. Arrows indicate the carbon atoms of deoxyribose that are joined by phosphodiester bonds to form polynucleotides.

(Fig. 3.2). The nucleotide monophosphates are abbreviated to AMP, CMP, GMP and TMP if containing ribose; or to dAMP, dCMP, etc. if containing deoxyribose. Uridine monophosphate (or UMP) is a component of RNA and is equivalent to dTMP in DNA.

Primary structure of DNA

The nucleotides are the individual building blocks for nucleic acids and are linked together in long strands by phosphodiester bonds to form polynucleotides. This involves the hydroxyl group of carbon-3 and the phosphate group of carbon-5 of the sugar (arrowed in Fig. 3.2, see above) of two adjacent nucleotides. This polymerization of bases is frequently denoted in shorthand form as in Fig. 3.3. The structure of the DNA polynucleotide sequence is further stabilized by forming a double-stranded structure with a complementary sequence through the pairing of bases. The nucleotides of guanine and cytosine form a stable base pair, as do adenine and thymine. The base pairs are stabilized by hydrogen bonding between residues and finally results in a structure consisting of two antiparallel polymeric strands.

In double-stranded DNA the base-pairing is mainly between G–C (Guanine–Cytosine) and A–T (Adenine–Thymine) (Fig. 3.4) and this

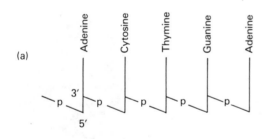

(b)   — — — pApCpTpGpA — — —

(c)   — — — pA —— C —— T —— G —— A — — —

Fig. 3.3 Shorthand notations for oligonucleotides.
(a) The vertical line denotes the carbon chain of the sugar with the base (adenine, cytosine, thymine, guanine) attached. The diagonal line indicates the phosphate link, at the top end the carbon-3' and at the lower end of the vertical line the carbon-5'. (b) Further abbreviation where the phosphate group is denoted by p; and when placed to the right of the nucleoside symbol the phosphate is esterified to carbon-3' of ribose; when placed to the left of the nucleoside the phosphate is esterified at carbon-5' ribose. (c) Further abbreviation by omitting p between the nucleoside residues.

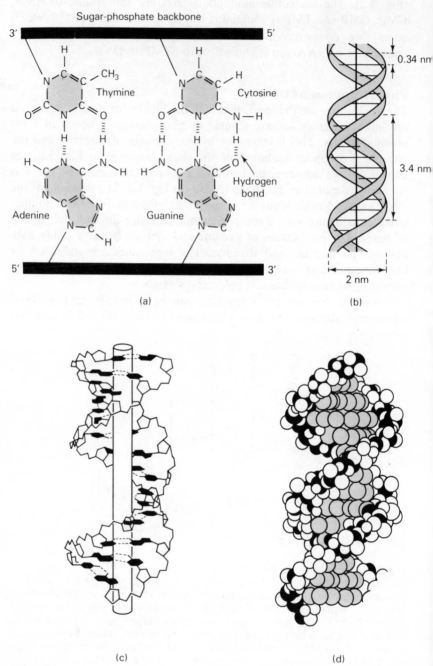

Sugar-phosphate backbone

Thymine

Cytosine

Adenine

Guanine

Hydrogen bond

(a)

0.34 nm

3.4 nm

2 nm

(b)

(c)

(d)

Fig. 3.4

explains an early observation by Chargaff that the sum of the purine bases in a nucleic acid molecule was the same as the sum of the pyrimidines. The notion of base-pairing was also a central point in the proposal of the double helix by Watson and Crick in 1958.

Helical structure of DNA

The first helical structure proposed was right-handed, consisting of two antiparallel strands stabilized by hydrogen bonding with phosphodiester bonds between the sugar residues forming the backbone (Fig. 3.4). From model-building studies, several parameters of the helix structure could be predicted. Confirmation of these predictions with regard to base pairs per turn of the helix and axial rise per base pair come from X-ray diffraction studies. Some of these parameters are shown for the common B-form and other proposed helical models in Table 3.1. The most common structure of the proposed helices (the B-form) is right-handed and contains both a major and minor groove. In this form the bases are paired almost perpendicular to the sugar-phosphate backbone of the helix. Each turn of the helix contains 10 base pairs.

Table 3.1 Different parameters of the DNA double helix

Structural form of DNA	Pitch (nm)	Residues per turn	Axial rise per base pair in Å	Inclination of base pair from horizontal
A	2.8	11	2.6	20°
B	3.8	10	3.4	0°
C	3.1	9.3	3.3	6°

Source: Adams, R.L.P., Burdon, R.H., Campbell, A.M., Leader, D.P. and Smellie, R.M.S. (1981). *The Biochemistry of the Nucleic Acids*. Chapman and Hall.

Other forms of the helix differ from the B-form in both the number of residues per turn of the helix and their pitch (Table 3.1). The differences found amongst the A, C, and D forms affect the grooves of the helix and whether the helix is contracted or elongated. For example, in the A-form the helix is stubby compared to the B-form, which results in the major groove of the A-form being much larger with a consequent reduction of

Fig. 3.4 Typical base-pairing by hydrogen bonding in the DNA double helix. (a) Normal base-pairing arrangements found in DNA; two hydrogen bonds are formed between adenine and thymine; three hydrogen bonds between cytosine and guanine. The most important consequence of base-pairing is that the order of bases in one chain automatically determines the order in the other complementary chain. Bonds in the nucleic acids showing (b) the helical twists and the helix parameters, (c) the helical twist and base-pairing arrangements and (d) the space filling model of the double helix.

the small groove. This structure also results in the base pairs being stacked sharply at an angle to the helix.

Although the helix in the double-stranded form is a stable structure under physiological conditions, it can be easily disrupted. The hydrogen bonds stabilizing the helix can be broken and the two strands of DNA separated. Heating the DNA or treatment with mild alkali or formaldehyde causes separation of the helix into two strands that can be followed spectroscopically.

If heat is used to dissociate the strands of the helix, a characteristic melting curve can be obtained by following the absorbance of the DNA at 260 nm with gradual increase of temperature. Under these conditions no increase in absorbance is observed until the transition temperature is reached. At this point the hydrogen bonds of the helix are broken down and the absorbance at this wavelength increases sharply (Fig. 3.5). The final melting profile obtained is characteristic of certain features of the primary structure of the DNA. If the primary structure of the DNA is fairly homogeneous with regard to distribution of G–C and A–T base pairs, a sharp transition is observed indicating a uniform melting of the helix. However, A–T pairs are melted more easily than G–C base pairs (because A–T base-pairing is with two hydrogen bonds, compared to

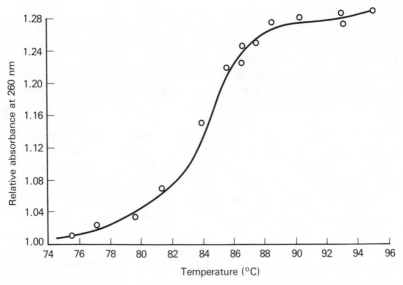

Fig. 3.5 A representative melting curve for a DNA double helix. Disruption of the DNA double helix with rising temperature produces an increase in absorbance at 260nm. This is sometimes called a 'melting curve' for DNA and its features can vary with the homogeneity of DNA used and its content, especially guanine and cytosine.

three for G–C), hence regions high in G–C residues melt less easily. An uneven distribution of base pairs throughout the DNA will lead to a less sharply defined transition point and more than one may be found.

After the helix has been disrupted it can reform again by re-annealing the two complementary strands. For example if the helix has been disrupted by heating, then slow cooling can cause it to reform. During the process of re-annealing, mis-matching may occur and long stretches of DNA may fold back on themselves giving rise to double-stranded loops within a single strand. These structures have been proposed to exist in native DNA.

The property of nucleic acids to re-anneal into double-stranded structures forms the basis of identifying genes by hybridization analysis. Even short sequences (of 15–20 bases) are able to anneal to complementary sequences under the correct experimental conditions. The process of annealing of two nucleotide sequences is known as hybridization and is fundamental to the method of Southern blotting described on p.59. The applications of this technique for detecting specific genes in the human genome or on particular chromosomes is described in Chapter 5.

Chromatin

A typical human chromosome contains a thread of DNA of approximately two metres in length if fully stretched. Yet this is packed into a nucleus of one hundredth of a millimetre in diameter. How can this packaging be achieved and yet still permit particular stretches of the DNA to function as genes?

The DNA within a chromosome is packed and organized by association with a variety of nuclear proteins. One of the main proteins associated with DNA are the histones, consisting of five major proteins. This family of proteins carry a net positive charge due to their amino acid composition; and their arginine and lysine residues interact strongly with DNA by forming stable salt bridges with the negatively charged phosphate group of the DNA backbone.

Under the electron microscope the DNA of chromatin appears to have a structure resembling a string of beads (Fig. 3.6). By gently digesting the chromatin with staphlococcal nuclease a basic unit of the chromatin structure is produced, the nucleosome (sometimes called the chromatosome).

The nucleosome consists of a core of eight subunits of histone proteins around which the DNA helix is tightly coiled. One of the histones (H1) is found on its surface, and may be associated with the entry and exit of the

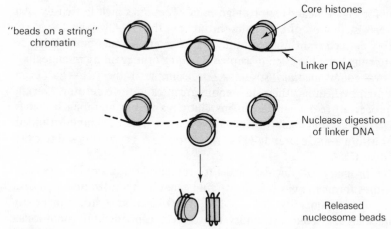

Fig. 3.6 A diagram of the supposed structure of polynucleosomes; which, after digestion with micrococcal nuclease are released from chromatin as beads (individual nucelosomes).

DNA from the nucleosome. The dimensions of the nucleosome are well-established and two turns of the helix can be wound around the outside of the histone core (Fig. 3.7).

The winding of the DNA helix around the nucleosome core compresses approximately 140 base pairs of about 600Å in length into a core particle of 100Å . Further packing may be achieved by organizing coils of nucleosomes into a solenoid-like structure. However, it is still unclear how these solenoid structures are organized to pack the genetic material within the chromosome. Some further complex looping or coiling must

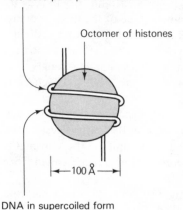

Fig. 3.7 A possible model for a nucleosome.

occur to increase still further the packing ratio (of the fully extended DNA length versus the chromosome length).

The nucleosomes isolated from chromatin all contain the same complement of histone proteins. However, differences are observed between nucleosomes due to the modification of the histones or the presence of non-histone proteins. Histones may be modified by acetylation or phosphorylation and this may possibly modify the activity of adjacent genes. Of the non-histone proteins, the high mobility group (HMG) proteins may be modified by phosphorylation, and fractions of chromatin enriched in sequences containing active genes may contain increased amounts of HMG proteins.

The structural properties of chromatin may thus be intimately linked to the differential action of genes. Two possible mechanisms involving structural changes in DNA are under current investigation. One is the possibility that regions of actively transcribing chromatin are unfolded and are more sensitive to digestion by the enzyme DNA-ase I (Fig. 3.8). Regions that have increased sensitivity to digestion by DNA-ase I have been mapped to regions adjacent to actively expressed genes. Secondly,

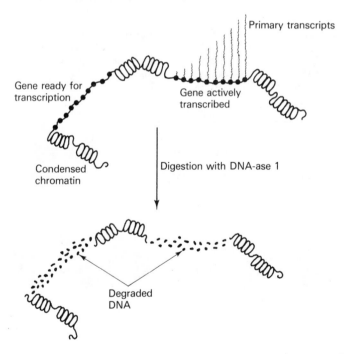

Fig. 3.8 DNA-ase hypersensitivity sites may occur close to actively expressed genes. Mild digestion of chromatin with DNA-ase 1 can degrade actively transcribing genes and potentially active genes.

the modification of cytosine residues in the DNA helix by addition of large hydrophobic groups such as methyl residues, may lead to local alterations in chromatin structure. Methylation of DNA has been proposed as a possible means of regulating gene expression by affecting the binding of DNA-associated proteins. However, both these ideas are still the subject for future research.

Gene structure and function

One of the central dogmas of molecular biology defines the direction in which information passes from the gene to protein. The steps are:

$$\text{DNA gene} \xrightarrow{\text{transcription}} \text{RNA message} \xrightarrow{\text{translation}} \text{Protein product}$$

Many of the details of how this process is accomplished and the basic mechanisms by which genes are regulated are now partly understood.

The basis of the process is that the DNA nucleotide sequence of the gene is faithfully copied as a nucleotide sequence in messenger RNA

Table 3.2 The genetic code. Sets of 3 nucleotides in mRNA are translated into amino acids corresponding to individual codons e.g. UUU is translated into phenylalanine and UCU into serine. The codons UAA, UAG and UGA are stop signals for the termination of translation. The AUG codon for methionine also serves as an initiator codon for the start of translation.

5'-OH terminal base	Middle base				3'-OH terminal base
	U	C	A	G	
U	Phe	Ser	Tyr	Cys	U
	Phe	Ser	Tyr	Cys	C
	Leu	Ser	STOP	STOP	A
	Leu	Ser	STOP	Trp	G
C	Leu	Pro	His	Arg	U
	Leu	Pro	His	Arg	C
	Leu	Pro	Gln	Arg	A
	Leu	Pro	Gln	Arg	G
A	Ile	Thr	Asn	Ser	U
	Ile	Thr	Asn	Ser	C
	Ile	Thr	Lys	Arg	A
	Met	Thr	Lys	Arg	G
G	Val	Ala	Asp	Gly	U
	Val	Ala	Asp	Gly	C
	Val	Ala	Glu	Gly	A
	Val	Ala	Glu	Gly	G

(mRNA), which can then serve as a template to build up the amino acid sequence of the protein. The genetic code provides the rules for the translation of the nucleotide sequence of the message into the amino acid sequence of the protein. The sequence of bases in the mRNA are read off serially in groups of three, a set of three nucleotides being called a codon. Each codon specifies one amino acid. The codon dictionary is presented in Table 3.2. It is evident that most amino acids are specified by more than one codon; thus the code is degenerate (e.g. leucine can be coded by CUU, CUC, CUA and CUG). However, there are differences in the frequency in which different codons specifying the same amino acid are used in individual cells for protein synthesis.

The matching of amino acids to the various codons of mRNA is achieved by a set of transfer molecules, called transfer RNA (or tRNA). These are RNA molecules of about 70–90 nucleotides long and act as carriers because they contain a sequence of three nucleotides (an anticodon) which is complementary to the codon of the mRNA. They will thus bind to the appropriate codon of the message, at the same time as carrying in the amino acid to be linked to the growing peptide chain on the ribosome.

The Wobble hypothesis
Because the code is degenerate many different tRNA species, recognizing different codons may still specify the same amino acid. However, the number of tRNAs is less than the number of codons, hence some tRNAs may recognize more than one codon. The explanation lies in the Wobble hypothesis. Only the first two nucleotides of the tRNA anticodon need to pair exactly with those of the codons in mRNA. The third nucleotide can pair to other nucleotides than its usual partner. Consequently the same anticodon can bind to two or three codons differing in the third base, although all specifying the same amino acid.

The gene
The classical idea of genes as discrete units of heredity, defined by recombinational events, were for many years regarded as a 'string of beads' along a chromosome. Later recognition that one gene made one protein (or peptide) allowed a definition of a gene in molecular terms. A gene is equivalent to a stretch of DNA coding for the amino acid sequence of a peptide. This is not necessarily a continuous stretch of DNA since in most genes of eukaryotes the coding sequence is interrupted by lengths of non-coding sequences, called introns.

The definition will not apply strictly to all genes because there are several examples where one gene can code for different proteins. This arises from differential processing of primary gene products to give different RNA molecules which are then translated into different proteins. Another complication is that in some bacteriophage genes (such as ϕ X 174), the use of different reading frames allows the same stretch of DNA to code for different proteins. However, these exceptions can still be accommodated in the original definition if it is accepted that different genes can overlap on the same stretch of DNA.

The definition must be further qualified in view of the fact that the number of genes in a cell is not equal to the number of proteins, since DNA does not just code for protein. Ribosomal RNA and tRNA are also copies from the nucleotide sequence of DNA contained in genes.

DNA organization in eukaryotes

Most of the DNA in the nucleus of higher organisms does not code for protein. The average mammalian genome contains about 3×10^9 nucleotides, enough to code for 1.5×10^6 different proteins (see Table 1.2, p.7), but only a fraction (less than one per cent) actually does so. The remainder of the DNA may have other functions such as the maintenance of complex structure and packing of DNA in chromosomes.

Repetitive DNA sequences

About 30 per cent of DNA in the eukaryotic genome consists of DNA sequences that are repeated many times. By contrast, most structural genes coding for protein are present as single copies. The repetitive elements are of two types: satellite DNA and interspersed repeated DNA.

Satellite DNA consists of tandemly repeated sequences in stretches of between 170–250 nucleotides long. They do not appear to be transcribed and are clustered in the region of heterochromatin associated with the chromosomal centromere. The sequences do not appear to be highly conserved during evolution, probably because their repetitive nature encourages duplication and deletion of large blocks of DNA during genetic recombination.

The second type of repetitive elements are dispersed randomly throughout the genome. They vary in length from several hundreds to several thousands of base pairs, and can be subdivided into different families. The relative abundance of these elements has so far defied explanation. They may be involved in the regulation of gene expression; or alternatively, since no phenotypic or evolutionary role has been yet found for them, they may be parasitic, and have been termed by some investigators as 'selfish DNA'.

The best characterized repetitive elements are those belonging to the Alu family. These elements were first isolated from the human genome and consist of short interspersed sequences of approximately 300 nucleotides long, which represent at least five per cent of the entire genome. About 60 per cent have a common cleavage site with the restriction enzyme Alu I. The Alu repeat family consists of closely related sequences and is the most abundant single class of DNA within the human genome. They appear to be randomly distributed throughout the genome and are found near all structural genes. Two Alu repeats have been described in the β-globin gene cluster in a region believed to be important in gene regulation. The Alu sequences can be transcribed and are found in both poly A^+ and poly A^- hnRNA fractions (heterogeneous RNA [hn RNA] is a diverse assortment of RNA molecules found in the nucleus, including a mRNA precursors.)

It has been suggested that Alu repeats may form part of the transposable elements of the genome. Prokaryotes and eukaryotes contain DNA elements several kilobases long that can move from site to site within the genome. They are called transposons and have short repeated sequences at each end. Since there are also short repeated sequences in the flanking region of Alu sequences, it is possible that they are also mobile and may explain their abundance and dispersal throughout the genome.

Eukaryotic gene structure

The view that genes are continuous stretches of nucleotides of DNA containing the coding sequences for a protein molecule, holds true for genes of prokaryotes, but does not apply to most eukaryotic genes. In these coding sequences (exons) are interrupted by long stretches of non-coding sequences (introns).

Introns appear to separate coding sequences for different domains of a protein. This may confer greater evolutionary advantage in eukaryotes since they provide potential sites for recombination leading to duplication or combination of useful protein domains. The collagen gene is an example of a gene which has arisen by duplication. The gene is 40 kb pairs long and its coding information is subdivided into at least 52 exons. The introns vary in length from 50–2000 base pairs. Many of the exons have an identical length of 54 base pairs and it seems likely that collagen genes have arisen from an ancestral gene by multiple duplications of a single genetic unit containing a 54 nucleotide exon. Later evolution of the exon sequences may have occurred by successive point mutations and by the addition or deletion of sequences.

Many eukaryotic genes are arranged as families, i.e. they are situated within a few kilobases of each other on the same chromosome. They have all presumably arisen by successive gene duplications. Clustered genes include those of the globin family, genes for HLA antigens, immunoglobulins and the interferon genes. The genes coding for apolipoproteins A-I and C-III of the human serum lipoproteins are also clustered and lie within 2.6 kb of each other. They both show homology in protein sequence and again, presumably arose by duplication from a common ancestor (Fig. 6.2).

Gene duplication has probably also given rise to a group of DNA structures called 'pseudogenes'. These are DNA sequences with strong homology to functional genes but are not active due to the accumulation of deleterious mutations that prevent expression.

The general structure of a eukaryotic gene is presented in Fig. 3.9. Apart from introns and exons, genes contain common flanking sequences required for efficient expression. These are promotors, enhancers, sequences for polyadenylation and capping of the 5′-end of the mRNA.

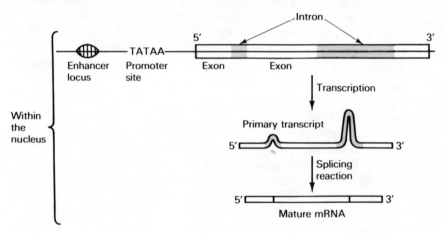

Fig. 3.9 Various structures of a eukaryotic gene and its transcription into RNA.

Control of gene expression

Differences between cell types are determined by differences in the proteins they produce. Much of the control of this appears to be at the level of transcription, but very little is known about the process in eukaryotic cells. In prokaryotes, regulatory proteins (such as inducers or repressors) may bind to specific DNA sequences (or operator sites) to modulate the binding of RNA polymerase and so activate or repress transcription of the adjacent gene. The best example of this is the control of the *lac* (lactose) operon of *E. coli*. The control of expression in eukaryotes is very much more complex, but may share similar features.

Transcription

The synthesis of a RNA molecule whose nucleotide sequence is an exact copy of the DNA sequence of the gene is termed transcription. DNA transcription is a crucial step in the transfer of informaton from DNA to protein. Although it is best understood in prokaryotes, where possible, details will be given for eukaryotic cells since this is more relevant to an understanding of molecular mechanisms in metabolic disease.

Briefly, in prokaryotes an enzyme, RNA polymerase, binds to a specific region of DNA, the promotor sequence, which is a signal for RNA synthesis is to begin. The polymerase unwinds the DNA helix and then the enzyme travels along the DNA template in a $5 \rightarrow 3'$ direction. The incoming ribonucleoside triphosphates pair with complementary bases on the DNA strand and are joined together by the action of RNA polymerase to form the RNA chain. The process continues until it encounters a punctuation sequence in the DNA, the termination signal, where the polymerase releases the newly synthesized RNA chain. The process is illustrated in Fig. 3.10.

The promotor is a site, usually on the $5'$-side of the gene, that binds RNA polymerase for the start of transcription; it also determines which of the two DNA strands in the gene is to be copied. The promotors of *E. coli* have been well characterized. The enzyme recognizes two sequences in the DNA strand located about ten and 35 nucleotides from the start of transcription (that is the first codon of the first exon). The DNA sequence at position ⁻10 from the start of transcription (called the Pribnow or TATA box) shows homology amongst a large number of bacterial and viral promotors. The prototype sequence is TATAAT where the first two and last nucleotides in the sequence are stringently conserved. Similar promotor-like sequences are found on the $5'$-side of many eukaryotic genes.

Enhancer sequences

The rate of transcription can be greatly influenced by DNA sequences distinct from promotor sites. These enhancer sequences were first identified in SV40 virus, and can involve DNA sequences lying immediately upstream or overlapping with the promotor. They greatly increase the transcription of SV40 even when they are removed from the promotor and reinserted thousands of base pairs away. The effect of these sequences has been strikingly demonstrated by measuring mRNA synthesis after transfer of structural genes into tissue culture cells. For example, when rabbit β-globin gene is transplanted into HeLa cells, little globin mRNA is synthesised, even though the gene contains a promotor. However, when SV40 enhancer sequences are inserted into plasmids containing the β-globin gene, mRNA production is increased 200-fold.

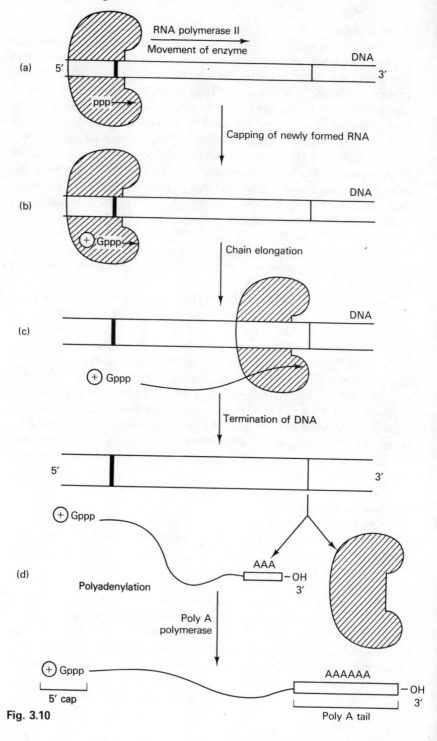

Fig. 3.10

Such enhancer sequences influencing gene expression have also been identified in the 5'-flanking regions of the human insulin and chymotrypsin genes. These sequences are located upstream of the promotors and have the property of increasing transcription of the gene in cells in which they are normally expressed.

Transcription in eukaryotes
Transcription of eukaryotic genes is far more complex than in prokaryotes. The essential differences are that in eukaryotes the primary transcript undergoes processing before the formation of mRNA. The coding sequences, or exons, of eukaryotic genes are interrupted by stretches of intervening DNA (introns) which are transcribed but not translated. The whole of the DNA sequence is transcribed and then the intervening sequences are spliced out, to leave the coding sequences in the mRNA. In addition, during transcription the RNA is covalently modified at one end. At the 5'-end a special base, usually 7-methyl guanosine is linked through a triphosphate group to the 5'-end of the mRNA. This cap may influence binding of mRNA to rRNA during the subsequent process of translation. At the 3'-end a long stretch of adenine nucleotides (the poly A tail) is added after transcription that may affect transport of the RNA from the nucleus into the cytoplasm. Up to 200 residues of adenine can be added at the 3'-end; and many eukaryotic mRNAs have sequence homology at about 11–30 nucleotides from the addition of the poly A tail. The consensus sequence is AAUAAA and is the only sequence homology found in the 3' non-coding region that could be a recognition site for enzymes involved in polyadenylation of the primary transcript.

There are three different RNA polymerases in eukaryotes, each of which transcribes different sets of genes. Polymerase I transcribes genes that make large rRNAs; polymerase II transcribes genes that code for cellular proteins; and polymerase III makes a variety of small stable RNAs such as tRNA and the small RNAs of the ribosome. These enzymes can be distinguished by their sensitivity to inhibitors such as cordycepin and α-amanatin.

The transcripts of polymerase II in the nucleus are called heterogenous nuclear RNA (hnRNA). Most of this is processed in the nucleus to mRNA, and before release to the cytoplasm is covalently modified by capping at the 5'-end, and polyadenylation at the 3'-end, as previously described.

Fig. 3.10 Transcription in eukaryotes. RNA polymerase II produces a transcript (or copy into RNA) from the DNA template (a,b). The transcript is immediately modified at the 5'-end with the cap structure ⊕ G ppp (b,c). The enzyme reads through the nucleotide sequence of the gene, making an RNA copy. Finally a polyA tail is added to complete the primary transcript (d).

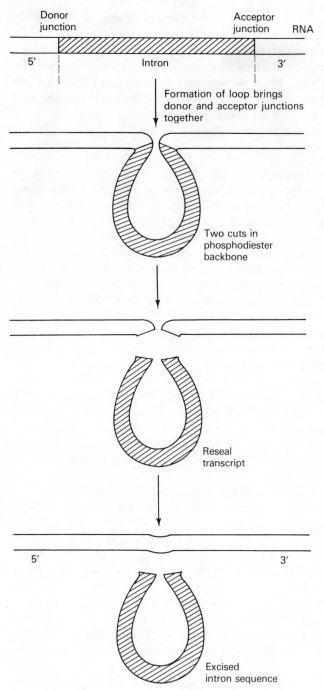

Fig. 3.11 Splicing out of introns during the processing of a primary RNA transcript, aided by ribonucleoprotein, leads to the introns forming loops. The chain is then cut at the donor and acceptor junctions and then rejoined.

Processing of primary transcripts

The primary transcripts are packed in ribonucleoprotein particles in which they are guided through the subsequent steps of mRNA processing. These transcripts (hnRNA) are unstable and short-lived and consequently comprise only a small fraction of total cellular RNA.

The average length of hnRNA is about 8000 nucleotides, which is much longer than the 1200 nucleotides needed to code for the average protein of 400 amino residues. The reason for the large difference in size is due to the presence of introns. These range in size from fewer than 100 nucleotides to 10 000 nucleotides. They differ from exons in that much of the nucleotide sequence can be altered without greatly affecting gene function. However, there are a few nucleotides at each end of the intron that cannot be changed without disrupting gene function. These conserved boundary sequences are believed to be signals for RNA

Primary transcript

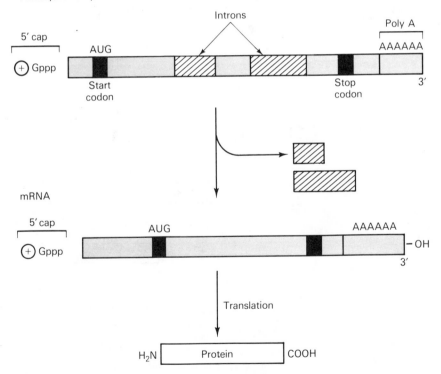

Fig. 3.12 Processing of the primary RNA transcript. The 5' cap structure at the 5'-end and polyA tail at the 3'-end are characteristic of eukaryotic mRNA. The primary transcript is larger than the mRNA due to the presence of introns, which are spliced out to yield the mature mRNA. The AUG codon is the start site for translation, and the stop codon signals the end of translation.

splicing (Fig. 3.11).

Enzymatic cleavage and restoration of the chain at these sites remove the introns intact – a process that must be precise since an error of even one nucleotide would alter the reading frame of the resulting RNA molecule and make nonsense of the message. Multiple intron sequences can be removed from a single RNA transcript and the process is illustrated in Fig. 3.12.

The splicing of primary transcripts usually joins the 5'-end of one intron junction to the 3'-end of the other intron junction. However, some RNAs can be processed in different ways to produce different mRNA codings for different proteins. The presence of introns thus makes for greater flexibility since different patterns in splicing can

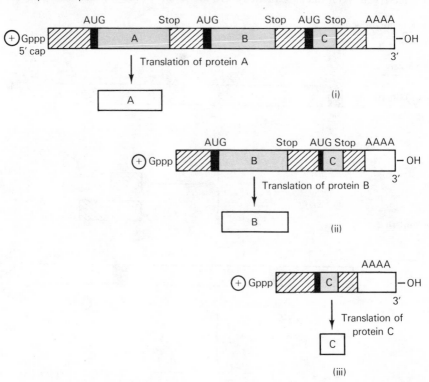

Fig. 3.13 Differential processing to give different mRNAs coding for different proteins. The primary transcript contains coding sequences for three proteins; A, B and C. The transcript can be spliced to remove sequences with adjacent introns to give three types of mRNA. The same cap site is used in each. Translation occurs from the 5'-end to the AUG stop codon, thus either protein A, B or C can be produced.

generate different proteins from the same primary transcript (Fig. 3.13). Differential splicing giving rise to different mRNAs has been shown to occur during transcription of the immunoglobuln, enkephalin and calcitonin genes.

Messenger RNA structure

Mature mRNA contains a 5′ cap site, coding sequences for translation into protein and a poly A tail. In addition, they contain untranslated sequences of varying length at both their 5′- and 3′-ends. The leader sequence at the 5′-end can vary from ten to 200 nucleotides. The leader sequence of prokaryotes contains a purine rich stretch of about ten nucleotides from the start codon. A complementary stretch of pyrimidine sequences is found at the 3′-end of ribosomal RNA. Shine and Dalgarno have proposed that these complementary sequences may be involved in the recognition site for the initiation of protein synthesis, since the 3′-end of the rRNA could bind to the 5′-leader sequence of mRNA to ensure that translation starts at the correct initiation codon (AUG). The leader sequence in eukaryotic mRNA may also be important in the regulation of translation. However, no regions of homology have been found amongst leader sequences of different mRNAs; and there are no complementary regions between the leader sequence of eukaryotic mRNA and rRNA.

Translation

The synthesis of protein involves three major components: the mRNA which carries the coded message, the tRNAs which select the amino acids specified by each codon in the mRNA, and the ribosomes which bring these components together to form the peptide bonds. Ribosomes are large multi-enzyme particles comprising one large and one small subunit and contain about 50 per cent RNA. They contain a groove that accommodates a growing polypeptide chain and a groove that accommodates the mRNA molecule. These cover a stretch of about 30 amino acids and 35 nucleotides. They contain sites for binding tRNA linked to the growing polypeptide chain and for incoming tRNA-amino acids. The joining of amino acids is catalysed by peptidyl transferase, which is also bound to the ribosome.

There are three distinct steps in protein synthesis:

1. Initiation, where the ribosome is bound to a specific initiation site on the mRNA and the tRNA attaches to the initiator codon. Regulation of translation usually occurs at this stage.

2. Elongation, where incoming amino acids are joined to the carboxy-terminus of a growing peptide chain until the termination codon is reached, then

3. *Termination* and release of the nascent polypeptide chain.

Any mRNA molecule could potentially be decoded in one of three ways, since differing intiation sites could give rise to any one of three different reading frames. Consequently precise initiation at the start codon is crucial for translation. The start codon in both prokaryotes and eukaryotes is AUG, which is also the codon for methionine. The AUG codon at the beginning of the message is recognized by a specific initiator tRNA carrying methionine, which invariably initiates the polypeptide chain. Methionine is found at the amino-terminus of all newly synthesized proteins. Since the AUG codon can be found at other sites in the message coding for methionine, selection of the correct AUG codon at the start of the message is also crucial.

The initiation process is complicated, involving a number of steps catalysed by proteins termed initiation factors. Two signals are required for initiation; one is the AUG codon and the other is a signal required for binding the mRNA to ribosomes. The Shine-Dalgarno sequences may serve this function in prokaryotes, but other types of interaction must be involved in eukaryotes. The 5' cap site may be part of the recognition signal. At least seven different initiation factors have been identified in rabbit reticulocytes which are required for binding of mRNA to ribosomes, binding of initiator tRNA and the joining of ribosomal subunits.

After chain elongation there are three codons to signal chain termination (UAA, UAG and UGA). Hydrolysis of the final peptidyl tRNA bond is then followed by release of the nascent polypeptide. With secretory and cell membrane proteins the nascent peptide contains an N-terminal sequence of about 20–40 hydrophobic amino acid residues. This amino acid sequence, the signal sequence, may be essential for the binding of polysomes synthesizing these proteins to membranes of the rough endoplasmic reticulum. Only peptides carrying these sequences are capable of being transported across the membranes of the endoplasmic reticulum. The polypeptides thread their way across the membrane as they are synthesized and the signal sequence is then spliced off the peptide chain. Signal peptide sequences have been detected in many secretory proteins, including apoprotein A-1, the precursor of insulin, prolactin and growth hormone. They are not found in intracellular proteins such as the globins. The other details of ribosomal synthesis of protein are not strictly relevant to the rest of the contents of this book and will not be dealt with further.

Further reading

Adams, R.L.P., Burdon, R.H., Campbell, A.M., Leader, D.P. and

Smellie, R.M.S. (1981). *The Biochemistry of the Nucleic Acids*, 9th edition. Chapman and Hall, London.

(A classical account of the subject.)

Bradbury, E.M., Maclean, N. and Matthews, H.R. (1981). *DNA Chromatin and Chromosomes*. Blackwell Scientific Publications, Oxford.

(An excellent general introduction.)

Kornberg, A. (1980). *DNA Replication*. Simon and Schuster, New York.

(A classical account of DNA and mechanisms for replication.)

Lewin, B. (1974). *Gene Expression*, Vol. 1. John Wiley and Sons, New York.

Stent, G.S. and Calender, R. (1978). *Molecular Genetics: An Introductory Narrative*. W.H. Freeman, San Francisco.

Szekely, M. (1980). *From DNA to Protein*.Macmillan Press Ltd., London.

(A specialist monograph.)

Watson, J.D. (1976). *The Molecular Biology of the Gene*, 3rd edition. Benjamin, Menlo Park, California.

Watson, J.D. and Tooze, J. (1980). *The DNA Story*. W.H. Freeman, San Francisco.

(History of recombinant DNA research: letters, addresses, essays and lectures.)

4

Background to cloning

A decade has now passed since the construction of the first recombinant DNA molecules. These are molecules in which DNA from different origins are ligated together covalently. Initially hybrids were formed from different drug resistance genes carried on plasmid DNA of bacteria; and later hybrids of bacterial drug resistance factors and toad genes for ribosomal RNA were synthesized. Shortly after these experiments a moratorium was declared suspending research into recombinant DNA which was followed in 1975 by the National Institute of Health (NIH) guidelines to control such work. Public and scientific concern regarding the safety of these techniques persisted for some time although they are now regarded as being safe when applied to the isolation of human genes. Very strict safeguards still apply to the genetic manipulation of microbiological pathogens.

This chapter is not a laboratory manual describing how these techniques are performed; it will mainly describe the aims, purposes and uses of such techniques and in some instances give examples of results. By such techniques one can now isolate any human gene for which there is a known product or assayable function. They depend on the ready availability of a large number of enzymes which break, modify, synthesize or join fragments of DNA; and the ability to isolate DNA molecules that can replicate autonomously from bacteria (e.g. plasmids) or yeast to act as vectors for such fragments.

Enzymes that break DNA molecules, the restriction endonucleases, were first suspected in the early 1950s, when it was noticed that phage (a bacterial virus) grown on one strain of *E. coli* failed to infect a different strain. It later became clear that the phage DNA was being broken down by enzymes in the *E. coli*. The host DNA was protected from such attack by methylation of certain nucleotides.

Restriction enzymes were first isolated in the early 1970s and now more than 150 are available from a number of biotechnology firms. A

Table 4.1 Some restriction enzymes and their properties

Microorganism	Abbreviation	Sequence of DNA cleaved (5′ → 3′) (3′ → 5′)
Escherichia coli RY13	Eco R1	G↓AATTC CTTAA↑G
Haemophilus influenza Rd	HindIII	A↓AGCTT TTCGA↑A
Haemophilus parainfluenzae	Hpa I	GTT↓AAC CAA↑TTG
Haemophilus parainfluenzae	Hpa II	C↓CGG GGC↑C
Providencia stuartii 164	Pst I	CTGCA↑G G↓ACGTC
Bacillus amyloliquefaciens H	Bam H I	G↓GATCC CCTAG↑G
Haemophilus aegyptus	Hae II	PuGCGC↓Py Py↑CGCGPu
Streptomyces albus G	Sal I	G↓TCGAC CAGCT↑G

characteristic of these enzymes is their recognition of a specific sequence of nucleotides in DNA where they will form a breakage point, and they usually cut within (or occasionally outside) this sequence. Examples of restriction enzymes and their properties are given in Table 4.1. Other enzymes used in genetic manipulation are presented in Table 4.2.

The main methods to be described are the extraction, labelling, synthesis and sequencing of nucleic acids; and then their cloning in different vectors.

Isolation of nucleic acids

DNA
Many studies in the 'new' genetics begin with the isolation of DNA from the human cells of patients and control groups. This is for an analysis of the genetic constitution of the parent cells. A convenient cell-type to use is the leucocyte; enough DNA ($\approx 200\mu g$) can be obtained from 10–20ml

Table 4.2 Some enzymes used in genetic manipulations

Enzyme	Uses
DNA polymerase 1	Converting single-stranded DNA molecules to double-stranded forms. Also used for 'nick-translation' of DNA to prepare radioactive probes for hybridization studies.
Reverse transcriptase	Synthesizing cDNA on a mRNA template. Also for conversion of single-stranded cDNA to double-stranded forms.
DNA ligase	Sealing single-stranded 'nicks' in DNA duplexes. Also for covalent linking of flush-ended DNA duplexes.
Restriction endonucleases (Type II only)	To cleave DNA duplexes at defined recognition sites.
DNA-ase 1	For limited treatment of double-stranded DNA to introduce nicks for nick translation.
DNA ligase	Sealing single-stranded nicks in DNA duplexes. Also for covalent linkage of flush-ended DNA duplexes.
Nuclease S1	For destroying single-stranded DNA, e.g. trimming away single-stranded ends after converting single-stranded cDNA to the double-stranded form.

of blood for analysis of about 40 genes or for the production of a genomic library. High molecular weight DNA is isolated from such cells by the following steps:

1. cells are lysed with a detergent and the nuclei collected by centrifugation;

2. the nuclei are disrupted by treatment with the detergent sodium dodecyl sulphate;

3. attached proteins are removed by treatment with a proteinase followed by phenol/chloroform extraction;

4. the DNA is recovered by precipitation with ethanol.

The DNA is usually 40–100kb in length and pure enough to be used in restriction enzyme digests or cloning experiments.

RNA

Since the majority of gene products are RNA molecules a study of the

RNA content of a cell can be used to assess gene activity; particularly whether genes are activated or repressed by hormones or dietary factors. The hormonal activation of a gene results in the production of a specific messenger RNA which can be assayed. The isolated mRNA molecule can also be used to make a DNA copy and so yield information on the coding sequence of the gene. Isolation of RNA is more difficult than DNA because of the widespread occurrence of RNA degrading enzymes within cells. The easiest methods rely on the rapid denaturation of cell proteins followed by selective precipitation of RNA. The partially purified RNA is then freed of protein by phenol/chloroform extraction.

A useful starting point is the intact polyribosome (a number of ribosomes strung together on a long mRNA molecule) from a specialized cell that contains in abundance the mRNA of interest e.g. the insulinoma cell to isolate mRNA for insulin. The steps for isolation are:

1. The cells are lysed in buffer containing inhibitors of RNA-ase and the nuclei removed by centrifugation.
2. The polyribosomes are then precipitated from the supernatant by addition of a high concentration of magnesium ions. These polysomes contain mRNA and many ribosomes with nascent protein attached (Fig. 1,4).
3. The mRNA is then isolated from these structures by column chromatography, often relying on the selective adsorption of special features of mRNA (such as their tail of polyadenines) onto complementary tracts of nucleotides attached to the support medium i.e. polyuridine or polydeoxythymidine.
4. Finally the bound mRNA is eluted from the column using low strength salt solutions.

To identify the mRNAs isolated an *in vitro* translation system can be used. This is a cell free extract (often from rabbit reticulocytes) with high rates of protein synthesis but without any endogenous mRNA. When the purified mRNA is added protein synthesis commences and the peptide products can be analysed by gel electrophoresis and autoradiography if radiolabelled amino acids are initially included in the cell free mixture. Antibodies can be used to precipitate specific peptide products of the *in vitro* translation system and so allow identification of a particular mRNA.

A disadvantage of these systems is that the usual modification of the initial protein product (cleavage of a propeptide, glycosylation, sialylation, etc.) does not occur. However, if the mRNA fraction is injected into a large cell, such as the toad oocyte, such post-translational modification does occur, and if radiolabelled amino acids are supplied to the cell the products can be analysed by gel electrophoresis and autoradiograpy.

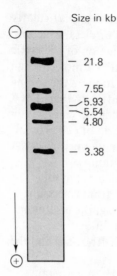

Size in kb

− 21.8

− 7.55
5.93
5.54
− 4.80

− 3.38

Fig. 4.1 Agarose gel electrophoresis of DNA visualized by ultra-violet light. The DNA bands are visualized by soaking the gel in solution of ethidium bromide which complexes with DNA by intercalating between stacked base pairs and photographing the orange fluorescence occurring on irradiation with ultra-violet light. The track contains phage DNA digested with the restriction enzyme Eco R1 and then electrophoresed on 1 per cent agarose gel.

Fractionation of nucleic acids

Having isolated DNA (or RNA) from cells it is often useful to fractionate them by size, since often only a particular sized molecule is of interest. Fractionation is usually performed by electrophoresis through slab gels of agarose. The molecules migrate towards the anode at a rate inversely proportional to the logarithm of their molecular weight. After separation on gels the dye ethidium bromide is used to stain the nucleic acid which then fluoresces when illuminated with ultra-violet light. A typical appearance of a gel photographed under ultra-violet light is shown in Fig 4.1.

An alternative method of fractionation which may be more convenient, if the nucleic acid is to be isolated, it to use sucrose density gradients in which the sedimentation rate in an ultracentrifuge is roughly proportional to molecular weight.

Labelling of DNA and RNA

In further studies with purified nucleic acids it is very useful to have them radiolabelled. They can then be used for hybridization studies with patients' nucleic acids after gel electrophoresis, and be detected by autoradiography. Labelling of DNA and RNA can be performed by attaching ^{32}P at the 5′-end from γ-^{32}P-ATP with the enzyme, T$_4$ polynucleotide kinase. Alternatively, the 3′-end of DNA can be labelled using the enzyme terminal transferase which attaches a ^{32}P dideoxyadenosine onto this end.

The method of 'nick-translation' uses DNA-ase to introduce nicks into the strand of DNA allowing a DNA polymerase to excise stretches of DNA and so serially move the 'nick' along one of the DNA strands. Radiolabelled nucleotides supplied in the reaction mixture then replace the missing nucleotide of the 'nick'. This usually includes ^{32}P-labelled α-CTP and may include other labelled nucleotides if a very high specific activity is required (Fig. 4.2).

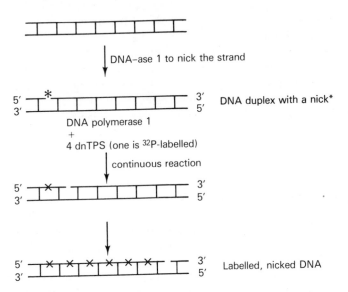

Fig. 4.2 Diagram illustrating nick translation of DNA. DNA polymerase I makes a 'nick' in a DNA chain as a starting point from which one strand of duplex DNA can be degraded, and replaced by resynthesis with new nucleotides.

There is a current trend away from the use of ^{32}P as a label in preference to non-radioactive systems. For some applications it may be possible to use nucleotides substituted with biotin which can be detected in an enzyme-linked immunoassay. Alternatively, fluorescent ligands may become of use.

Synthesis of polynucleotides

Two types of synthesis are currently in use: the synthesis of short stretches of nucleotides up to 50 base pairs in length (oligonucleotides); and the synthesis of DNA whose sequence is complementary to mRNA sequences (i.e. cDNA).

Synthesis of oligonucleotides

There are two major uses for these oligonucleotide sequences. They can be used to initiate DNA synthesis on fractions of mRNA to make a complementary copy. For example, if the oligonucleotide sequence codes for a unique stretch of the peptide of interest then it may preferentially hybridize with its mRNA to prime the synthesis of cDNA. Secondly, the oligonucleotide can be used as a probe to screen a cDNA library (see p.54) to identify clones that carry complementary sequences. Oligonucleotides can be synthesized in cycles, each of which adds one or two bases to the growing chain. Several chemical reactions, such as the phosphotriester method, can be used to join nucleotides together. By the addition of several nucleotides at certain points in the cycle it is possible to synthesize complex mixtures of oligonucleotides. It therefore becomes possible to synthesize a pool of oligonucleotides representing all possible triplets coding for a short stretch of amino acids in a peptide of interest. This can then be used as a probe to identify DNA sequences coding for that peptide in a cDNA library, and thus allow isolation and identification of the gene.

Synthesis of cDNA

DNA sequences complementary to mRNA can be built up if one starts with a short single-stranded primer. The primer can be a stretch of oligo-thymidines which will bind to the poly-adenine tail of messenger RNA; or be a mixture of oligonucleotides designed to be complemenary to a predicted RNA sequence derived from the known amino acid sequence of the peptide of interest. The flow-sheet for the method is shown in Fig. 4.3. Briefly, the enzyme reverse transcriptase will copy the mRNA into a complementary strand of DNA. The mRNA is removed by treatment with alkali and a second strand of DNA is synthesized on the first strand using a fragment of the enzyme DNA polymerase of *E. coli* (the Klenow fragment), which is devoid of exonuclease activity.

The second strand synthesis can be primed by a hairpin loop that appears at the 3'-end of the initial cDNA strand. The resulting double-stranded cDNA can be trimmed with an enzyme, SI nuclease, to remove the hairpin loop, and the resulting blunt-ended molecule can be ligated into a plasmid or phage vector for cloning. There are various ways of inserting the double-stranded cDNA into a vector: one is to add artificial Eco RI sites to either end and then ligate the fragment into the Eco RI site of a plasmid or phage; the other is to add a tail of 10–20 deoxycytidines to the cDNA and a similar number of deoxyguanidines to the cleaved vector. When the two sets of molecules are annealed, and then repaired, the vector can transform a host cell for replication.

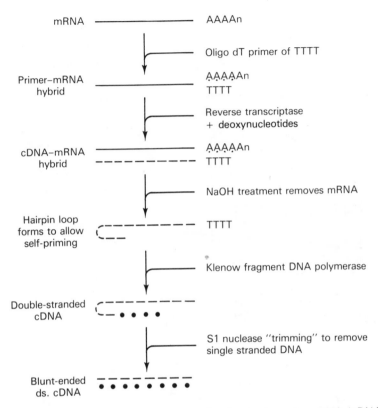

Fig. 4.3 Flow diagram for the synthesis of complementary DNA (cDNA) from messenger RNA (mRNA).

DNA sequencing

The final test to identify a DNA molecule is to examine its sequence. A gene is finally identified by seeing if its nucleotide sequence codes exactly for the amino acid sequence of the peptide product. Two methods of DNA sequencing are in common use with the potential to analyse up to 1000 base pairs per day. The chemical method of Maxam and Gilbert involves the isolation of a fragment of DNA labelled at one end with ^{32}P. The fragment is then subjected to a series of random but base-specific cleavages to produce a series of products. These are separated by size on very thin polyacrylamide urea gels at high voltage and the labelled fragments detected by autoradiography. Many unlabelled fragments are also produced but do not interfere with the autoradiography. A typical example of such a sequencing gel is shown in Fig. 4.4; the DNA sequence can be read off from the ladder of each of the base-specific tracks

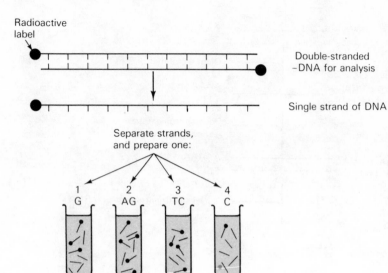

Radioactive
label

Double-stranded
–DNA for analysis

Single strand of DNA

Separate strands,
and prepare one:

| 1 | 2 | 3 | 4 |
| G | AG | TC | C |

Chemicals in tubes destroy one or two
of the four bases and breaks strand at these
sites variable creating a set of fragments of different
sizes.

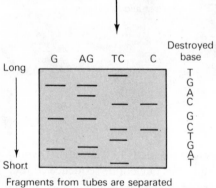

Fragments from tubes are separated
by size on gel electrophoresis and visualized
by autoradiography.

Sequence of strand read from below

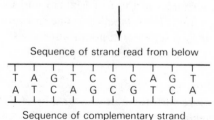

Sequence of complementary strand

Fig. 4.4 DNA sequencing by the method of Maxam and Gilbert.

starting from the bottom of the gel.

The second method, developed by Sanger and Coulsen, is more biological and involves the cloning of the DNA fragment into single-stranded filamentous virus called M13. A short DNA primer is used to initiate synthesis of a copy of the inserted DNA whose sequence is desired. However, this synthesis is interrupted randomly but specifically by labelled dideoxynucleotides (a chemical analogue of deoxynucletide) present in the reaction mixture which stops the growth of the chain at any point where the natural deoxynucleotide should be introduced. The resulting set of reaction products are analysed in the same gel system as the Maxam and Gilbert method, and the DNA sequence can be read off.

Cloning

If large amounts of a purified DNA molecule are required, for example as a reagent to perform hybridization studies with the human genome, it can be obtained by growing it in a suitable vector in a host cell, usually in bacteria or yeast. Construction of such a vector involves the introduction of the segment of DNA to be cloned into an autonomously replicating vehicle such as a bacterial plasmid or a bacteriophage (Fig. 4.5). The technical details of how the DNA of interest is inserted into the vector need not be considered here. The hybrid molecule of plasmid plus foreign DNA is now introduced into a suitable host, such as *E. coli*, by treatment of the cells with calcium chloride. *E. coli* containing recombinant molecules of DNA can be selected by the loss of antibiotic resistance of the host if the inserted DNA interrupts a gene coding for resistance, say to tetracycline. Alternatively, a colour indicator system can be used which depends, for example, on the interruption of the galactosidase gene by the inserted DNA. In this system 'wild-type' colonies develop a blue colour, whereas recombinants remain white because they cannot metabolize the indicator incorporated in the agar gel to its coloured form.

The main differences in the available vectors are in the lengths of DNA which can be accommodated and the efficiency with which recombinants can be obtained. If a phage (or cosmid) vector is used instead of plasmid, larger amounts of DNA can be packaged into the head of the phage, often followed by a higher efficiency of transformation of the *E. coli* host, and subsequent yield of the DNA molecule of interest.

Gene libraries and banks

The two terms are synonymous and refer to a large collection of individual fragments of DNA growing in a suitable host such as *E. coli*.

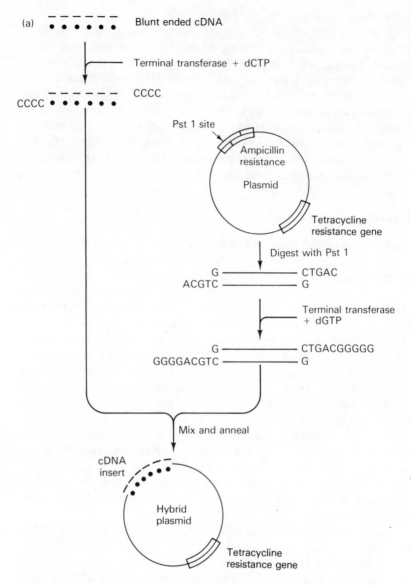

Fig. 4.5 Flow diagram for cloning DNA: (a) a preparation of hybrid plasmid and (b) transfection *E. coli* with hybrid plasmid.

A genomic library is a collection of fragments of nuclear DNA; a chromosomal library is a collection of fragments derived from a specific chromosome; and a cDNA library is a collection of expressed sequences derived from the total mRNA population of a cell.

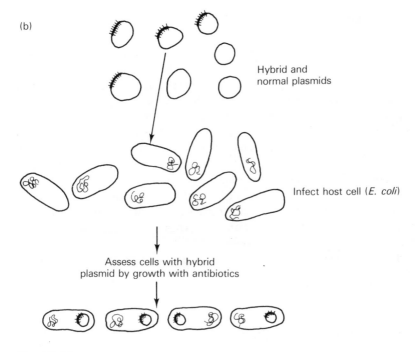

(b)

Hybrid and
normal plasmids

Infect host cell (*E. coli*)

Assess cells with hybrid
plasmid by growth with antibiotics

Fig. 4.5 (b)

cDNA libraries

Most tissues will contain more than 10 000 different mRNA species derived from active genes. Often 10–20 species are present at about 0.5–2 per cent of the total mRNA; 1000 species may be present at 0.01–0.5 per cent and more than 9000 present at less than 0.01 per cent of the total. To ensure capture of the rarest species in the library a large number of independent recombinant molecules must be generated by the methods described in the section of cDNA synthesis (p.48). The task can be made simpler by choosing a specialized cell where the mRNA of interest is present in abundance (10–20 per cent of the total mRNA). For example, globin mRNA can be obtained from reticulocytes; insulin mRNA from tumours of the β -cells of the pancreatic islets (insulinomas). Thus only a small number of recombinants need to be analysed to detect the sequence of interest. Otherwise cDNA libraries containing 10^5 to 10^6 independent recombinants are needed to ensure representation of the rarest species of mRNA in the cell.

cDNA libraries allow the easy identification of expressed sequences which can be used directly as probes to study gene organization, although much more fine detail of the organization of a single gene can be obtained after it has been isolated from a genomic library.

Genomic libraries

In the case of genomic or nuclear DNA there are more than 3×10^6 kb in the human genome and is thus clearly more complex than a mRNA population. The DNA can be handled in much larger pieces than single gene-sized fragments as derived from mRNA. The nuclear DNA can be partially digested with restriction endonucleases to obtain a random population of fragments which can be selected for different size ranges by fractionation on agarose gels or sucrose gradients. Fragments of 15–20 kb can be inserted into bacteriophage vectors and pieces between 35–40 kb can be accommodated by cosmid vectors. In the first case more than 800 000 and in the second more than 300 000 recombinants must be analysed to ensure detection of single copy sequences. Genomic sequences are important for the study of the number and position of intervening sequences (introns) and the types of regulatory sequences at the 5'- or 3'-end of the gene.

Both libraries can be stored as stocks of phage or *E. coli* (containing hybrid plasmids) so that the whole library may be present in a few microlitres of culture medium.

Identification of recombinants

The problem here is to pick out from a library of possibly more than 10^6 recombinant DNA molecules, the one that is of particular interest for further study. The procedure is to make a copy of the library growing on agar plates and then transfer it to a nitrocellulose membrane (Fig. 4.6). When the DNA of the *E. coli* colonies is denatured by alkali and the filter baked in an oven, the DNA remains tightly bound to the membrane and represents a copy of the DNA sequences present on the original agar plates. There are then various methods to identify the patch of DNA of interest; and so go back to the colonies of the original library to grow it up in large batches. Once isolated a cDNA clone can be used to select the corresponding genomic clone from a genomic library.

Oligonucleotide probes

If a small stretch of the protein sequence is known an oligonucleotide can be designed and synthesized which will hybridize to the cDNA baked onto the nitrocellulose filter. The probe is labelled with ^{32}P and hybridized in solution to the filter-bound DNA. Adjusting the temperature and salt contents of the solution for washing off unbound probe allows the removal of all the mismatched hybrid pairs, whilst the correctly matched sequences remain bound together. The sequences in

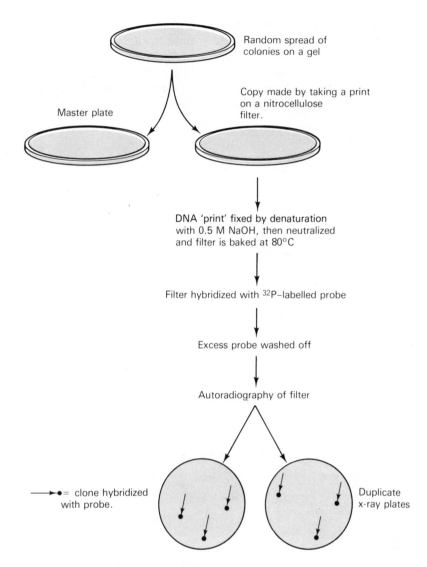

Fig. 4.6 Flow diagram for identification of recombinants by hybridization methods. Recombinant clones hybridize with probe (arrowed clones); probe can be mRNA, synthetic DNA or an antibody.

the probe mixture which are not exactly complementary to the sequences for which they were designed, do not usually pair up exactly with other DNA fragments in the library (on the filter) and so the number of false-positives is usually small.

Immunological methods for detection

If a protein sequence is not available to make an oligonucleotide probe, a clone can still be identified if there is an antibody to the protein. The method here is to use the DNA bound to the filter to hybridize with its corresponding mRNA from a sample of total mRNA. The specific mRNA can be eluted from the filter and translated in an *in vitro* translation

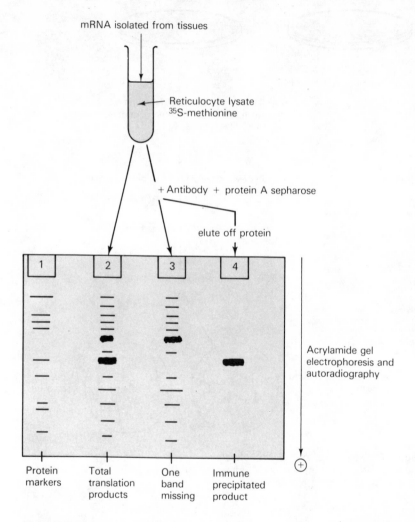

Fig. 4.7 *In vitro* translation; mRNA from tissue is translated into proteins using a rabbit reticulocyte lysate to supply ribosomes, enzymes etc. Incorporation of ^{35}S-methionine into newly made proteins allow visualization after gel electrophoresis and autoradiography. Specific identification of a protein can be made by antibody precipitation or elution techniques as shown in tracks 3 and 4.

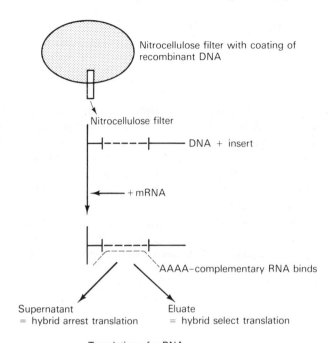

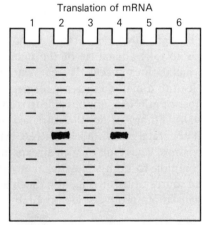

Track 1 = protein markers for molecular weights

Track 2 = total mRNA translation into proteins

Track 3 = hybrid arrest translation (one missing mRNA
bound to disk)

Track 4 = hybrid select translation (bound mRNA eluted for
translation).

Fig. 4.8 Flow diagram for identification of recombinants by hybridization
methods.

system (Fig. 4.7). The products of translation can be identified by immunoprecipitation and so characterize the original DNA bound to the filter (Fig. 4.8).

Expression vectors

In some cases the vector is designed to allow expression of the inserted DNA, so that the host cell synthesizes a part of the normal product of the gene which may be detected by the use of immunological screening. A copy of the library is now made on cyanogen bromide activated paper (to fix the protein products firmly by covalent bonding); and the bound proteins are then hybridized with the discriminating antibody for localization, usually by autoradiography. When a clone has been identified that yields a positive signal (i.e. produces a protein that hybridizes with the antibody) it can be selected from the original agar plate and grown to abundance. The DNA insert of the vector can be mapped with a series of restriction enzymes, and its DNA sequence can be determined. The DNA sequence can be compared with any of the amino acid sequence of the protein to confirm isolation of the correct clone.

Induction/repression methods

A useful way of detecting foreign DNA in vectors without prior knowledge of their structure is to take advantage of the induction of mRNA levels by hormones or metabolites in cells. If treatment of a cell or tissue with a hormone can lead to a marked increase (or decrease) in the level of one or a small number of mRNAs, it is possible to study these alterations by making a cDNA library from the enriched mRNA population and then screen it separately with labelled RNA extracted from the stimulated or resting tissues. The result of such an experiment is that there are many signals common to both states but that there are some specific for the stimulated source of tissue (Fig. 4.9). Such mRNAs can be isolated and their translation products identified by hybrid selection studies.

Similar types of experiments can be used to isolate clones containing cDNA which are characteristic of certain tumours or leukaemias. These neoplastic cells may be expressing genes that are not normally expressed in the healthy cell. The main disadvantage of this technique is that it only compares major differences between tissues and does not positively identify which mRNA species are involved. Differences between normal and diseased cells (such as dystrophic muscle cells or cells from patients with cystic fibrosis) should be amenable to this approach, to identify any unusual genes that may be activated in the disease state.

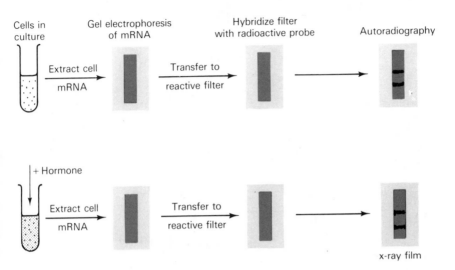

Fig. 4.9 Schematic results of an induction experiment examining changes in mRNA levels. Note two strongly hybridized bands appear from cells treated with hormone compared to untreated cells, suggesting that the hormone stimulates mRNA synthesis.

Gene analysis: Southern blotting

This technique, named after its inventor Dr. E. Southern, is currently one of the most useful for clinical studies, enabling an assessment of the genetic determinants of metabolic disease. A direct study of the fine structure of the relevant gene; a study of polymorphic variants; or a study of nucleotide alterations that act as genetic markers, can all be performed with this method. Usually leucocyte DNA is digested with a battery of restriction enzymes and fractionated according to size on agarose or polyacrylamide gel (Fig. 4.10). The DNA is visualized by staining with ethidium bromide and fluoresced by ultra-violet light to ensure completeness of digestion. The DNA on the gel is denatured with alkali, neutralized with Tris buffer, and transferred by capillary flow of a high salt solution to a nitrocellulose filter – the blotting process. The DNA is firmly bound to the filter by baking. The filter now carries a 'print' of the DNA from the gel which can be hybridized to a labelled gene probe. This can be a cloned DNA sequence or a synthetic oligonucleotide. If the complementary sequence is present in the human genome in one or a few copies a simple pattern of bands emerge after autoradiography. A restriction map of the sequence can be constructed by a series of suitable single or double enzymic digests.

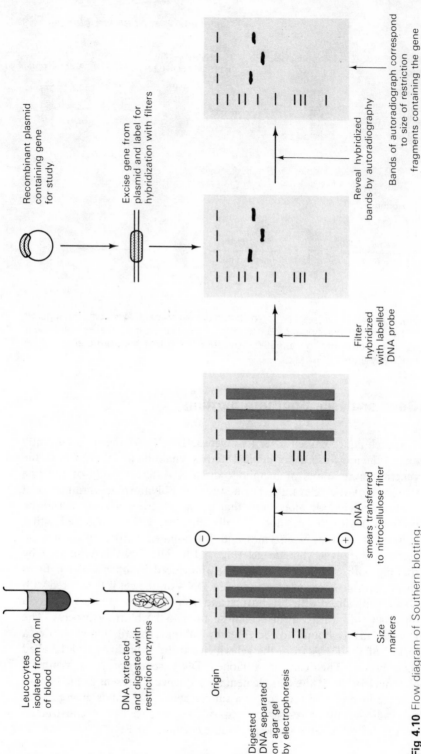

Fig 4.10 Flow diagram of Southern blotting.

Leucocytes isolated from 20 ml of blood

DNA extracted and digested with restriction enzymes

Digested DNA separated on agar gel by electrophoresis

Origin

Size markers

DNA smears transferred to nitrocellulose filter

Filter hybridized with labelled DNA probe

Recombinant plasmid containing gene for study

Excise gene from plasmid and label for hybridization with filters

Reveal hybridized bands by autoradiography

Bands of autoradiograph correspond to size of restriction fragments containing the gene

If an abnormal gene function is suspected the map in the affected individual can be compared with that of the normal. This technique can detect insertions or deletions of DNA of greater than 50–100 base pairs. In this manner deletions or insertions around the insulin gene and point mutations in the apoprotein C-III gene have been identified.

A more common use for Southern blotting is in the detection of restriction fragment length polymorphisms (RFLPs). These are the consequence of base rearrangements which create or destroy a recognition site for a restriction enzyme and are inherited in simple Mendelian fashion. These changes often may have no effect on protein synthesis or gene function and have been estimated to occur once in every hundred bases throughout the genome. These changes occur less frequently within the protein coding region or regulatory sequences of the gene. However, the method of Southern blotting can generate far more allelic variants than is possible by a study of protein polymorphisms. It is now possible to take a gene which has no protein variants associated with it and in a relatively short time discover several DNA variants at that locus (Fig. 4.11). Such DNA variants may be in linkage disequilibrium with base variation within the coding region of the gene and can have diagnostic value. The first example of this was the sickle cell mutation in the β-globin gene of people of West African origin. In this case the sickle cell mutation (coding for glutamine instead of valine) in the β-globin is linked to a restriction site mutation more than 2000 base pairs on the 3′-end of the β-globin gene (Fig. 4.12). More usually, the linked polymorphism is not associated with a particular allele and cannot be used for diagnosis. However, the polymorphism can be used as a linked genetic marker in family studies to follow the inheritance of the adjacent gene through family relatives.

A technique of increasing importance is the use of synthetic oligonucleotides to detect single base changes that may contribute to a genetic disorder. An oligonucleotide (about 19 bases long) is synthesized to be complementary to either the normal or mutant sequence and the conditions of hybridization chosen such that the normal probe only binds to the normal sequence (or the mutant probe only to the mutant sequence). This technique has been used in the diagnosis of a number of thalassaemias and sickle cell disease.

A number of pitfalls in the use of Southern blotting should be noted. Apart from technical problems (poor activity of restriction endo-nucleases, incorrect hybridization buffer, poorly labelled gene probe, etc.), there are often problems of interpretation. Anomalous bands running behind the normal position may be a new variant or it may be due to incomplete digestion of the genomic DNA by the restriction enzyme, producing an artefactual large band. The variable methylation

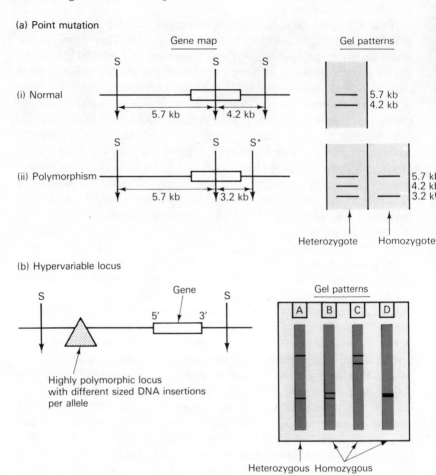

Fig. 4.11 Two types of DNA polymorphisms revealed by Southern blotting. (a) This map illustrates a hypothetical gene digested with the restriction enzyme (S) together with the blotting patterns after gel electrophoresis of the DNA fragments. The normal allele is shown in (i), the polymorphic allele in (ii), and the new S site marked by *. When occurring with the normal allele three bands are produced on Southern blotting; when occurring in homozygous form only two bands are formed of 5.7 and 3.2 kb in size. (b) The hypervariable polymorphism; two bands produced per diploid genome vary in size depending on DNA insertions of the polymorphic locus.

of restriction sites can also alter the banding pattern and so confuse the interpretation of polymorphisms. Contamination of genomic DNA with plasmid DNA can lead to strong artefactual signals if the probe itself is carried in plasmid DNA (due to plasmid-plasmid interaction). Unexplained artefactual bands appear in the region of the normal bands

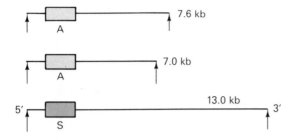

Fig. 4.12 Linkage of the sickle cell mutation in the ß-globin gene with a restriction site polymorphism. Above are three types of restriction fragments produced with Hpa1 and hybridized with the globin gene. A and S are normal and sickle ß-globin genes; the 13.0 kb fragments are found with more than 80 per cent of the globin S genotype, but only in approximately 10 per cent of healthy controls.

and although they often differ in signal intensity and shape they can appear very similar to the usual band. Frequent replication with a 10-fold increase in restriction enzyme and family studies to track the inheritance of the anomalous band can help to clarify these anomalies.

RNA analysis: Northern blotting

Finally, blotting procedures can be used in analysis of RNA. Northern blotting is the RNA equivalent of Southern blotting. The RNA is now fractionated on an agarose gel and transferred by blotting to nitrocellulose. A radiolabelled DNA probe allows the detection of the corresponding RNA sequence bound to the nitrocellulose. If RNA is extracted from nuclei the sizes of the precursors can be determined (Fig. 4.13). An estimate of the abundance of the mRNA can be made and the response to hormonal or metabolic stimuli can be followed.

S1 nuclease mapping usually involves the hybridization of nuclear RNA or mRNA with a fragment of genomic clone under conditions that favour the formation of DNA–RNA hybrids rather than DNA–DNA hybrids. Any single-stranded DNA that has not hybridized with the RNA is subsequently digested with a nuclease S-1 that is specific for single-stranded DNA. Surviving DNA has been protected from digestion by hybridization with its complementary RNA. This DNA can be analysed on a gel to determine its size or can be subjected to DNA sequence analysis to determine the exact ends of binding to the RNA. This method can determine the site of the 5'-end of RNA, the presence of introns at the 5'-end of genes, or the site of insertions/deletions in the RNA molecule.

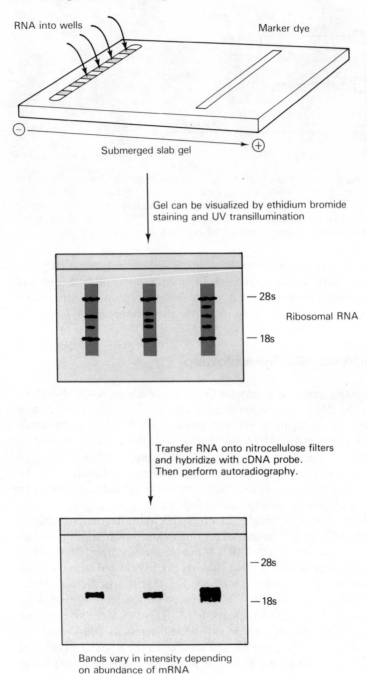

RNA into wells

Marker dye

Submerged slab gel

Gel can be visualized by ethidium bromide staining and UV transillumination

— 28s

Ribosomal RNA

— 18s

Transfer RNA onto nitrocellulose filters and hybridize with cDNA probe. Then perform autoradiography.

— 28s

— 18s

Bands vary in intensity depending on abundance of mRNA

Fig. 4.13 A flow diagram of Northern blotting.

Further reading

Maniatis, T., Fritsch, E.F. and Sambrook, J. (1982). *Molecular Cloning: A Laboratory Manual*. Cold Spring Harbour Laboratories, New York.

Old, R.W. and Primrose, A.B. (1981). *Principles of Gene Manipulation*. Blackwell Scientific Publications, Oxford.
(A text concentrating on basic methodologies.)

Williamson, R. (1981). *Genetic Engineering*, Vols 1–4. (Vol. 1: Essays on cDNA libraries; antenatal diagnosis of haemoglobinopathies, expression of cloned genes. Vol. 2: Essays on gene evolution, genomic libraries, use of restriction enzymes and gene cloning in yeast. Vol. 3: Essays on plasmid and M13 cloning vectors, expression of cloned genes in eukaryotic cells, a list of cloned eukaryotic genes. Vol. 4: Essays on DNA engineering, applications to characterization and expression of polypeptide hormones, expression of eukaryotic genes in *E. coli*.) Academic Press, London.
(An excellent series of introductory volumes to the listed topics written mainly for postgraduates in biochemistry.)

5

Genetic polymorphisms

It is readily apparent that a description in conventional terms of the pathology of a variety of common metabolic diseases, such as atherosclerosis, hyperlipidaemia, and diabetes mellitus (and their complications) is inadequate as regards pathogenesis. What is being described are the gross macroscopic end-products of the disease state, but the initial biochemical events which are responsible for the development of the condition and its complications are being ignored. As pointed out in Chapter 1, some progress has already been made in the detailed biochemical analysis of some rare inborn errors of metabolism which turn out to have clear-cut enzymatic defects as their basis (see Table 5.1); where a simple underlying genetic defect leads to Mendelian inheritance of the disease in families. However, it is very likely that the more common metabolic diseases arise not from simple enzyme defects but from more complex errors in metabolic regulation involving either the rates of induction or repression of enzymes or receptors; or from errors in the regulatory properties of enzymes or transport proteins. The inherited basis for these diseases may not be simple structural gene mutations but instead relate to common polymorphic genetic variants that confer susceptibility or liability for an individual to develop disease when exposed to a particular environmental condition (such as excess dietary loads of carbohydrate or lipid). This chapter will consider the types of genetic variants that occur; their appearance in populations; and their possible associations wth disease.

Gene mutations

A gene contains a sequence of DNA that codes for a particular protein or RNA molecule that is used by the cell. A typical structure of an eukaryotic gene is shown in Fig. 3.9 (see p.32).

To recapitulate, the important features to note are:

1. A promotor site at the 5'-end of the gene usually occurs within 30 nucleotides of the start of the coding region. The promotor site often includes the consensus sequence of nucleotides of TATAA. Other regulatory sequences such as operator and enhancer loci may occur that alter regulation of gene expression by hormones or other regulatory metabolites.

2. The coding sequence contains the segment of DNA that directly codes for the RNA and protein products. The coding region is often (but not always) interrupted by stretches of DNA called introns which are transcribed but not translated.

3. The 3'-end of the coding region where a stop codon acts as a termination signal for the end of protein synthesis.

4. A variable sequence after the stop codon that does not appear in the final gene product but contains a signal sequence that is involved in binding enzymes for the polyadenylation of the primary transcript (see p. 35);

5. the end of the gene is somewhat vaguely defined as the site where polyadenylation of the gene product (hnRNA) commences.

A gene (considered as a long sequence of DNA nucleotides, usually more than 1500 base pairs in length) has many sites where the DNA sequence can be varied to produce mutations. Various patterns of change in the DNA sequence can be considered and fall into two main categories: point mutations and sequence rearrangement mutations. They can occur anywhere along the gene involving regulatory sequences, coding sequences, intervening sequences, etc., and will have quite different effects on gene function depending on their exact location. If the mutation takes place in a germ line cell it may be transmitted to offspring and become a heritable trait. If it occurs in a cell not destined to form gametes, i.e. a somatic cell, its effects will be limited to the individual and the change is termed a somatic mutation.

Point mutations

These are the simplest cases where there is an alteration of a single nucleotide in the DNA sequence. A nucleotide base can be inserted, deleted or substituted by another purine (adenine or guanine), or by a pyrimidine base (cytosine or thymine). The effects depend on the exact location of the alteration and can be:

1. In the coding part of the gene. Consider the following example that uses the three letter English words to represent the codons:

THE FAT C̆AT ATE THE BIG RAT

If the nucleotide C is removed the information content becomes:

THE FAT ATA TET HEB IGR AT

and clearly the message is scrambled and the resultant protein likely to be

Table 5.1 Features of some inborn errors of metabolism

Condition	Deficient enzyme	Clinical features
Phenylketonuria	Phenylalanine hydroxylase	Mental retardation, reduced hair and skin pigmentation.
Galactosaemia	Galactose-1-phosphate uridyl transferase	Early cataracts of the lens. Failure to thrive.
Fructose intolerance	Aldolase B (liver enzyme)	Hypoglycaemia, failure to thrive.
Lactose intolerance	Lactase (intestinal)	Failure to hydrolyze ingested milk, chronic diarrhoea starting after birth.
Glycogen storage diseases:		
Type I (von Gierke's disease)	Glucose-6-phosphatase	Enlargement of the liver and kidney, no storage in muscle, hypoglycaemia and growth retardation.
Type II (Pompe's disease)	α-,4-glucosidase	Glycogen accumulation in most tissues, especially the heart.
Type III (Forbe's disease)	Amylo-1,6-glucosidase	Accumulation of an abnormal glycogen.
Type IV (Andersen's disease)	Amylo (1,4 $\rightarrow$ 1,6)-transglucosidase	Abnormal glycogen accumulates in the liver, leading to cirrhosis.
Type V (McArdle's syndrome)	Phosphorylase (muscle)	Glycogen accumulates in muscle.

non-functional. If one substitutes an A at this site the message becomes:

THE FAT AAT ATE THE BIG RAT

The insertion suppresses the effect of the deletion by restoring most of the sense of the sentence and only one amino acid of the resultant protein is likely to be incorrect. By itself, however, the insertion will again scramble the message, e.g.

THE FAT ACA TAT TET HEB IGR AT

However, a nucleotide substitution does not always lead to an amino acid substitution because many triplets may code for the same amino acid. However, a different rate of synthesis of a normal protein may

Table 5.1 (cont.)

Adrenogenital syndrome	Steroid 21-hydroxylase	Virilization in females; .the external genitalia are masculinized, but internal genitalia are normal. Early fusion of bony epiphyses and short stature.
	Steroid IIβ-hydroxylase	Hypertensive form of congenital adrenal hyperplasia with clinical virilization –many patients showing hypertension.
	3β-hydroxysteroid dehydrogenase	Decreased synthesis of all adrenal steroids to give symptoms of adrenal insufficiency.
Goitrous cretinism (one type)	Iodotyrosine deiodinase	Gross enlargement of the thyroid with severe hypothyroidism due to defective deiodination of thyroid hormone precursors during synthesis.
Favism	Glucose-6-phosphate dehydrogenase	May develop acute haemolytic reaction after eating fava beans.
Congenital nonspherocytic haemolytic anaemia (one type)	Pyruvate kinase (erythrocyte)	Chronic haemolytic anaemia

result because of preferential codon usage by tRNAs during ribosomal assembly of amino acids into the nascent peptide.

2. In the intervening sequence. Since the majority of the intervening sequences of DNA, after transcription into RNA, are spliced out during processing of the primary transcript, nucleotide alterations may not have much effect on the gene product. However, at two sites, at either end of the intron (at intron–exon junctions) a nucleotide change can affect the way in which the intron is removed from the primary transcript. This is because there are preferred sequences bordering each end of the intron that may act as recognition sites for splicing enzymes to cleave at this site. Preferred sequences at either end are:

AG GUA – – – – – – – – – G GAC

splice site   splice site

Alterations here can result in abnormal splicing with the next splice sequence down- or upstream being used instead. This will result in an abnormally sized mRNA producing a defective protein, either longer or shorter than the normal protein.

3. In regulatory sequences. The same considerations apply, deletions, insertions or substitutions can occur but now the effect may be on the rates of synthesis or induction of a normal protein by regulatory metabolites such as steriod hormones. Thus, if the mutation affects the promotor site it may impair the binding of RNA polymerase for the initiation of gene transcription and reduced amounts of the protein will result. If the mutation affects the operator sites it may impair or facilitate the binding of a regulatory metabolite or protein and affect the rates of induction (or repression) of the gene-product. Transcriptional mutants have been recently found to occur in the regulatory sequences close to the β-globin gene, and impair synthesis of this product. Depending on the site of the nucleotide change in relation to the regulatory binding region, many variable effects could ensue.

4. At critical codons. Some codons act as signals for the start or termination of translation. For example, UAA, UAG or UGA are signals for chain termination, so if a point mutation alters such a triplet the resulting mRNA may code for a larger protein than the normal messenger and the protein product may be non-functional. Correspondingly, if a mutation occurs within the coding region to create a new UAG or UGA codon then the resulting protein will terminate prematurely and again will produce a non-functional protein.

5. At flanking sequences. All types of mutations can occur in the flanking regions of genes and although they may not affect the regulation of gene expression they can provide a wealth of new genetic markers to track the inheritance of the adjacent gene in family studies.

Mutations producing sequence rearrangements

These are grosser changes affecting segments of a gene or even large blocks of genes involving the loss, addition, inversion or displacement of DNA sequences. Their effects, like point mutations will depend on their exact location, whether in coding, regulatory, intervening or flanking sequences. There are a few major types of alterations:

1. Deletions.

A length of the genome is missing. Using small-case letters to represent genes or segments of approximately 100 nucleotides, the change appears as:

abc⁞defghi⁞jklmn → abcjklmn

where the sequence between the dotted lines is eliminated.

2. Inversion.
Here a segment of DNA is rotated from the 5′ → 3′ to 3′ → 5′ orientation:

abcdefghijklm → abcdefg mlkjih

3. Duplication.
Part of the genome is repeated:

abcdefghijkl → abcdabcdefghijkl

Such a repeated segment is called a tandem duplication because the new segment is adjacent to the original sequence. However, the duplicated sequence may appear elsewhere on the same chromosome or on another chromosome. Complete duplication of a gene, and then independent evolution of the two genes can give rise to families of proteins all derived from a common ancestral gene, e.g. the apolipoproteins have amino acid sequence homology to suggest they have derived from a common ancestral gene and arisen by a series of gene duplications (see p.16 for evolutionary implications).

4. Translocation.
Part of a chromosome is transferred to another, usually with reciprocal exchange of material.

Chromosome 1   abcdefghijkl ———————————→ abcdefghIJKL
Chromosome 2   ABCDEFGHIJKL ——————————→ ABCDEFGHijkl

These sequence rearrangements can have much more drastic effects on gene function than point mutations as they are more likely to interfere with the functional regions of the gene.

Examples of insertion/deletion and point mutations around the insulin gene are given in Chapter 7, p.108; and examples of point mutations in the region of the lipoprotein genes are described in Chapter 6, p.93.

Genetic polymorphisms

Mutations, as described in the previous section, are a fundamental way of altering the genome structure, and in some instances can produce a deleterious change in gene function. Such mutations will gradually become eliminated from the gene pool of the population under the influence of natural selection on the resulting phenotype. However, occasionally a mutation will arise that may have some selective advantage over the common allele, and may gradually increase in frequency to the point of permanent fixation in the population. When the frequency of the uncommon variant occurs to an appreciable extent that cannot be accounted for by new mutations (arbitrarily taken as more than one per cent), it is called a polymorphic variant. A genetic polymorphism is therefore the occurrence in the same population of two or more alleles at one locus, each occurring at an appreciable frequency and not accounted for by new mutations. The new variant may in fact be spreading through the population (i.e. be transient) or may be in equilibrium with the 'wild-type' allele (i.e. be a balanced polymorphism).

Genetic polymorphisms constitute a basic component of heriditary variation in natural populations on which evolutionary forces operate. A polymorphic variant which is at a minor selective disadvantage and may be declining in frequency, can become a selective advantage if the prevailing environmental conditions alter slightly. This therefore provides a means by which populations can evolve in different directions. In general, the greater the genetic variation inherent in a natural population, the greater the opportunities for evolutionary change.

The methods for detecting genetic polymorphisms have been described in Chapter 4. Briefly, genomic DNA is digested with particular restriction enzymes that cleave specific sequences and reveal the polymorphism by producing different sized fragments of DNA including the same genomic sequence. The variation in fragment size can be produced by mutations at the recognition site for restriction endonucleases, or by sequence rearrangements close to these sites. The genotype of an individual can be determined by the procedure of 'Southern blotting', as described on p. 59 and Fig. 4.10 (see p. 60).

Many genes have now been examined for adjacent polymorphisms. It has been calculated that one in every hundred nucleotides may be variable, making the extent of DNA polymorphisms much greater than that observed for protein polymorphisms as detected by gel electrophoresis. Gel electrophoresis of proteins requires that the polymorphic variants contain charge differences and so be easily separable in an electric field; substitution by neutral amino acids may not be revealed. On the other hand, DNA polymorphisms can be detected if:

1. The mutation directly affects a recognition site of a restriction endonuclease, either creating a new site or abolishing an old one. In either case a different sized DNA fragment will be produced (e.g. Fig. 4.12 p. 63). Over 150 restriction enzymes are available each with different nucleotide-sequence specificities and each enzyme is of potential use for detecting new polymorphisms. This is providing a wealth of new genetic markers for clinical studies.

2. The fragment of DNA produced by the restriction enzyme contains

sequence rearrangements within it. A good example of this is the highly polymorphic locus at the end of the insulin gene containing tandem arrays of an oligonucleotide repeat sequence. This makes a DNA fragment cleaved by the restriction enzyme Bgl1 highly variable in length when hybridized to the insulin gene probe.

From a preliminary analysis (human genomic probes have only been available since the mid-1970s), there is clearly a large amount of genetic polymorphism in human populations. Some of this polymorphism may be impermanent in the population representing a transient phase of molecular evolution. The rarer of the variant alleles could be in the process of increasing or decreasing in frequency, either under the influence of natural selection or by random genetic drift. Alternatively, the polymorphism may be permanent, i.e. be in equilibrium with the common form. The rare alleles may even be older than the evolutionary process that produced the species. How such alleles have remained in the face of selection and genetic drift is clearly a matter of great theoretical and practical interest.

Maintenance of polymorphisms

Several mechanisms have been proposed that may operate to maintain genetic polymorphisms in a natural population. Most of them have been explored theoretically and some have been subjected to rigourous experimental research. The three simplest mechanisms are heterozygous advantage, frequency dependent selection and random genetic drift. In the former the heterozygotes possess some selective advantage over the two homozygous genotypes. The advantage may be manifest as superior viability, fertility or fecundity of the individual; or a longer reproductive life. As a result the heterozygotes show superior fitness and leave relatively more offspring than other genotypes. Both alleles are passed on to succeeding generations and the polymorphism is maintained, but at the expense of creating homozygous genotypes of inferior fitness. Frequency dependent selection, on the other hand, involves a situation where the fitness of a genotype increases as its frequency declines. Consequently the genes composing this type are reproduced in relative excess when they become rare in the population. A trivial example of this may be preferential selection of a mate for unusual features, such as blue eyes and red hair! As the phenotype becomes rare it would be at a selective advantage for reproduction.

There are also other less well-studied mechanisms. Density dependent selection occurs when the fitness of the genotype is related to its population density; and this could maintain a polymorphism under certain conditions.

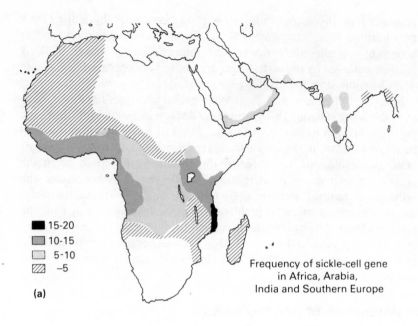

15-20
10-15
5-10
−5

(a)

Frequency of sickle-cell gene
in Africa, Arabia,
India and Southern Europe

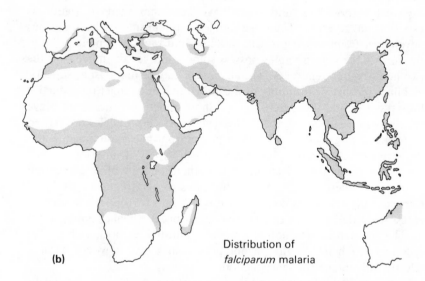

(b)

Distribution of
falciparum malaria

Fig. 5.1 Frequency distribution of the sickle cell gene and the occurrence of malaria. (From Alison, A.C. (1961) In *Genetical Variation in Human Populations*. Pergamon, Oxford.)

Heterozygous advantage

This is probably the most widely quoted method of maintaining a polymorphism. When the heterozygote is superior in fitness to both homozygotes then a larger proportion of heterozygous offspring survive to reproduce and both alleles are consequently maintained in the population.

The best example of this is the allele coding for sickle cell haemoglobin. This is a point mutation of the β-globin gene which codes for glutamic acid instead of valine. Subjects who are homozygous for this mutation possess red cells that undergo sickling and aggregation, particularly at low oxygen tensions. The disease presents as a chronic haemolytic anaemia with superimposed acute crises of vascular thromboses occurring anywhere in the body. This can lead to splenic infarcts, avascular necrosis of the femoral heads, cerebral thrombosis, etc. and is usually precipitated by infection or hypoxic episodes. The heterozygote is usually normal although he is making both sickle and normal (or adult) globin variants. Under extreme conditions of low oxygen concentrations the red cells collapse into their characteristic sickle shape and can lead to thrombosis.

The gene coding for sickle haemoglobin is present at high frequency among many populations of Africa and Southern Asia (Fig. 5.1) despite

Table 5.2 Some evidence that heterozygotes for sickle cell haemoglobin are protected from the effects of malaria from the incidence of sickle cell trait among African children whose deaths could be attributed to malaria. Note only one child died from malaria with the sickle cell trait, whereas 23 would be expected to die if no selective advantage was confered by the trait.

Locality	Deaths due to malaria	Number with sickle cell trait	Incidence of sickle cell trait in the population	Expected number with sickle cell trait if no selective differential
Uganda (Kampala)	16	0	0.16	2.6
Congo:				
Leopoldville	23	0	0.235	5.4
Luluaborg	23	1	0.25	5.7
Ghana (Accra)	13	0	0.18	2.3
Nigeria (Abadan)	29	0	0.24	7.0
Totals	104	1		23.0

Source: Harris, H. (1980). *Principles of Human Biochemical Genetics*. Elsevier, Holland.

its apparent selective disadvantage due to the increased mortality of the homozygotes. For many years the reasons for this were unclear until it was realized that red cells or heterozygotes (SA genotype) for the sickle globin gene were less likely to be infected by the malarial parasite, *Plasmodium falciparum*, than normal cells (AA) which are homozygous for adult globin. Some typical results supporting this theory are presented in Table 5.2. They indicate that heterozygotes are less likely to be infected with the malarial parasite and also that any infection is likely to be less severe. The balancing force maintaining the sickle globin gene in the population appears to be protection from the hazards of malaria, i.e. there is a negative disease association with the heterozygous form. The reason why red cells that contain sickle globin are less easily parasitized by *P. falciparum* than normal cells is not clearly understood but may be related to the fact that red cells containing the parasite may adhere to the walls of small blood vessels whilst the parasite matures. In such situations the oxygen tension may become low and the red cells start to assume their sickle shape, and then become phagocytosed by macrophages. The parasite may thus be destroyed before it reaches maturity and so does not reproduce to infect more red cells.

Frequency-dependent selection

A balanced polymorphism can occur if the fitness of a genotype is related to its frequency. For example, if the fitness of a variant genotype increases as its frequency in the population declines, there will be an increase in the relative proportion of the alleles composing this genotype in the next generation. Conversely, if the fitness declines as the frequency increases the trend will be reversed. Although frequency-dependent selection has not been demonstrated in human populations, it has been shown to operate in experimental animal populations, mainly involving situations such as competition between phenotypes for limiting nutrients; or differential mating preferences.

Although heterozygous advantage and frequency-dependent selection are the simplest methods for maintaining segregating alleles within a population, they are not the only selective mechanisms. More complex systems such as natural selection acting in different directions (diversifying selection); or changing selective forces on a phenotype during geological time could also maintain a polymorphism (see Chapter 7, p.112). Finally, some polymorphisms may be selectively neutral.

Random genetic drift

It is probable that most DNA polymorphisms are selectively neutral and their frequency changes in populations due to random genetic drift. A special example of this may be the increase in frequency of a rare genetic variant in a localized population due to the 'founder' effect. This can occur after a severe reduction in population size, and subsequent re-expansion from a few 'founder' genotypes, some of which may contain a rare allele that now becomes more frequent in that population. It can be due to immigration of a 'founder' genotype into a sparsely populated locality and then spread by differential reproduction. A good example of this is the gene for the rare metabolic disease Variegate Porphyria, which was probably introduced into S Africa by a Dutch immigrant in 1688 and has consequently spread in the white and black population there, achieving a frequency of about 300/100 000 births. It has probably spread by the founder effect despite the undoubted selective disadvantages that must attach to this genotype.

As previously described, genetic variability is a prerequisite for evolutionary change in populations, and mutation is the ultimate source of this variability. Useful mutations are stored in the gene pool of a population as genetic polymorphisms. Some of these polymorphisms may become deleterious due to a subsequent change in environmental conditions and become associated with disease processes. Deleterious polymorphisms are the price the species pays for possessing useful ones and in the long-run such genetic variability is a major factor enabling the population to adapt to changing environmental conditions in the future.

Disease association studies

The relationship between polymorphic systems and disease in man has been studied for many years. Initial observations were with polymorphic protein systems; and since the red cell group polymorphism (A, B, O) was one of the first systems to be described in 1900 by Landsteiner, disease associations were first sought here. The most obvious associations were found between the ABO groups and some forms of malignant disease, particularly of the gastrointestinal tract. Many other associations were reported (with duodenal ulcer, peptic ulcer, pernicious anaemia), but the increased risk of the disease state in persons with the relevant blood group was hardly greater than for those with other blood groups, being sometimes up to twice as common. Thus these polymorphic variants were clearly not applicable for diagnosis, prognosis or assistance in understanding the genetics of these diseases. Much more useful information was obtained between polymorphisms of the HLA system and associations with such diseases as leukaemia, Hodgkin's lymphoma, rheumatoid diseases (e.g. ankylosing spondylitis) and autoimmune diseases (myasthenia gravis, hyperthyroidism, insulin-dependent diabetes, etc), although very few of these have been of diagnostic value. An informative review of this system is in Bodmer (1978).

DNA polymorphisms

The first of the metabolic diseases studied for polymorphic variants was non-insulin dependent diabetes using the human insulin gene probe. A full description of these studies is given in Chapter 7, p.109. Other diseases, atherosclerosis, hypercholesterolaemia and hypertriglyceri-daemia, have quickly followed. In general, those diseases are worth studying which have a known or suspected hereditary element, and where a DNA probe is available for any gene that might be expected to be involved in the aetiology of the disease. Thus for diabetes mellitus, the insulin and insulin-receptor genes might be implicated; in the hyperlipidaemias some (or all) of the apolipoprotein genes may be involved. Diseases with a marked inherited component are likely to show the strongest associations with DNA variants; and pedigree studies for linkage between the DNA variants and manifestation of the disease should be performed. However, it should be noted that some diseases which were believed to have no obvious genetic mode of inheritance have revealed very startling associations with HLA antigens. An often quoted example is ankylosing spondylitis and its correlation with HLA B27, where over 90 per cent of Caucasian patients possess this antigen, compared to a general frequency of less than ten per cent in most Caucasian populations.

To recapitulate and expand the ideas of p.8, DNA probes can be used for at least four types of genetic studies:

1. A direct study of the fine structure of any gene by restriction enzyme mapping where an abnormal gene product is suspected to influence the aetiology of the disease. Good examples are the insulin gene mutants in some types of non-insulin dependent diabetes mellitus producing an insulin with impaired biological activity.

2. A study of DNA polymorphic sites adjacent to the relevant gene that may either affect some aspect of regulation of gene expression; or provide a marker for the affected gene to allow its identification in affected family members in a pedigree analysis. The use of a linked polymorphism in tracking a disease specific gene throughout members of an affected pedigree is illustrated schematically in Fig. 5.2

3. A study of DNA polymorphic sites adjacent to the relevant gene that may be in linkage disequilibrium with other, hitherto unsuspected, disease specific genes close to this locus, and may help in their eventual identification, and;

4. To study the arrangement of gene clusters, where genes involved in

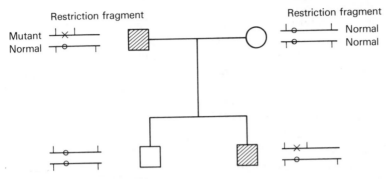

Fig. 5.2 Use of nonspecific DNA polymorphisms adjacent to a disease locus to track its transmission through a pedigree. A restriction site polymorphism is used to track a mutant gene (x) in a pedigree. There are two cutting sites (⊢⊣) for the restriction enzyme close to the mutant gene, but only one is close to the normal gene (o). The difference in size of the fragments can be easily detected on Southern blotting and allows identification of offspring to whom the mutant gene has been transmitted.

a particular aspect of metabolism may occur closely together on the same chromosome. Good examples of this are the β-globin gene cluster on the short arm of chromosome 11 involved in oxygen transport; and the apoprotein A1-CIII gene cluster involved in lipid transport.

Problems in design of studies: Lod scores

There are many problems in the design, statistical analysis and interpretation of studies using DNA probes. Some of these are now considered.

Definition of clinical groups.
The common metabolic diseases are a particularly heterogeneous group of disorders where multifactorial aetiologies are to be expected as the rule rather than the exception. If a search is to be made for genetic determinants, the groups of patients must be clearly defined and made as homogeneous as possible with regard to clinical diagnostic features before undertaking the genetic analysis. Many of these diseases (non-insulin dependent diabetes, the hyperlipidaemias) have a very variable age of onset before the diagnosis can be established with certainty. This can be partly corrected by the proper selection of controls to be age-matched.

Control groups

These must be carefully selected with regard to age. If the control group is two decades younger than the experimental group, and the disease does not normally appear before middle-age, it is quite possible that some of the control subjects will go on to develop the disease. It will therefore not constitute a good control group since potential diseased subjects are included. DNA polymorphisms appear to have a very variable distribution throughout racial (and possibly geographical) groups; so the controls must be matched for race and preferably geographical locality. Since the hereditary component of some of these diseases is an increased susceptibility to an environmental factor (such as dietary loads of carbohydrate or animal fats), control groups should ideally be exposed to similar environmental conditions.

Family groups

Although many diseases have a genetic component they may not exhibit familial clustering because the co-inheritance of several genes may be required for full disease expression. Useful information may still be obtained. A very instructive example, previously quoted, is the strong association of ankylosing spondylitis (not generally considered as an inherited disease) with HLA antigen B27. Perhaps other weakly familial diseases, like atherosclerosis, will be found to have strongly associated genetic markers.

Technical problems

Apart from the general technical problems of cloning and identifying gene probes, another major problem is the artefactual production of bands during hybridization studies. These can be very misleading as it is sometimes difficult to know if an abnormal sized fragment produced from the patient's genome is genuine or artefactual. Repetition of digests and a family study to see if the abnormal band appears in the first degree relatives in an expected Mendelian manner can help to elucidate these points.

Statistical analysis: Lod scores

Tests of association between disease and presence of a polymorphic variant are usually assessed by a chi-squared test of significance. Linkage disequilibrium can produce weak associations, but can lead on further to a search for more disease-specific genes in the vicinity. Genetic linkage between disease and a polymorphic variant can be supported in some studies by pedigree analysis. Briefly, the aim here is to analyse families for the distribution of the disease throughout the members and relate this to the distribution of the genetic marker. If the genetic marker always segregates with affected members and is never observed in unaffected members, this is suggestive evidence for genetic linkage. For example, on inspection of the imaginary family of Fig. 5.3, three generations are available for study in which diabetes mellitus is segregating (solid-filled symbols). L and S represent genetic markers such as the length of the polymorphic locus close to the insulin gene, described on p.106. Subject II-1 is diabetic inheriting L from his father (who is also diabetic) and has handed on L to III-1 and III-4 who are both diabetics (i.e. two non-recombinants). Subject II-2 is not diabetic and inherited an S. allele from her mother and father; she has handed on S to III-2 and III-3 who are non-diabetics. However, II-1 has handed on L which came to him on a paternal chromosome to III-5 who is not diabetic, which either argues against linkage of disease to marker, or the possibility that recombination has occurred.

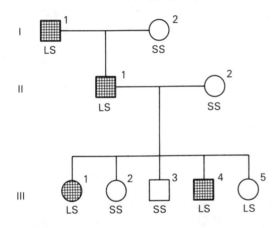

Fig. 5.3 Hypothetical pedigree to illustrate linkage and Lod scores. In this pedigree, diabetes (solid symbols) is segrating and individuals are genotyped for a marker (L and S alleles); see the text for full explanation.

The probability of linkage is tested statistically by Lod scores. Lod scores (meaning the logarithm for the odds for linkage versus odds for non-linkage) represents the weight of the evidence given by a family for or against linkage, and is usually tested at various recombination fractions (Θ) ranging from 0.00 – 0.45. The score is calculated as a logarithm so the values from different families in which the same disease segregates can be added together. Autosomal linkage can be considered established when in a collection of families the sum of the Lod scores at any value of Θ reaches + 3. If the sum of the Lod scores at a given value of Θ is less than − 2 then linkage is ruled out. The most informative families are those of three generations in which the parental genotypes are established of whom one with the disease is homozygous for the genetic marker and the other heterozygous for the genetic marker. Two generation families are also useful if there are many siblings with variable distribution of the disease amongst them. Lod scores are helpful in two ways: they show when the family data collected is sufficient to establish linkage and they enable data from different families to be pooled. They are usually calculated from computer programmes, or can be laboriously performed by hand; interested readers should consult Emery (1976) for the details of such calculations.

Further reading

Bodmer, W.F. (1978). *The HLA system. British Medical Bulletin*, Vol. 34, No. 3. The British Council.
(A collection of papers on the implications of HLA for clinical disease.)
Cavalli-Sforza, L.L. and Bodmer, W.F. (1971). *The Genetics of Human Populations*. W.H. Freeman and Co., San Francisco.
(A largely mathematical treatment of the subject.)
Emery, A.E.H. (1976). *Methodology in Medical Genetics: An Introduction to Statistical Methods*. Churchill Livingstone, Edinburgh.
(Methods used for the analysis of pedigree data.)
Hartl, D.L. (1980). *Principles of Population Genetics*. Sinauer Association, Massachusetts.
(A largely mathematical treatment of this complex subject.)
Lewin, B. (1980). *Gene Expression: Eukaryotic Chromosomes*, Vol. 2. John Wiley and Sons, New York.
(Very comprehensive account of eucaryotic genes – extensively referenced.)
Lewin, B. (1983). *Genes*. John Wiley and Sons, New York.
(A teaching text on genes and gene function – very good.)
Suzuki, D.T., Griffiths, J.F. and Lewontin, R.S. (1981). *An Introduction to Genetic Analysis*. W.H. Freeman and Co., San Francisco.
(An excellent undergraduate textbook on modern genetic analysis.)

6

The hyperlipidaemias

The hyperlipidaemias are a common group of metabolic disorders characterized by an abnormal accumulation of different lipids in plasma. The major lipids are cholesterol and triglyceride which are transported amongst tissues by the plasma lipoproteins. The plasma lipoproteins vary greatly with regard to size, lipid composition and peptide content. In general, each particle is a complex macromolecular aggregate consisting of a predominantly non-polar lipid core surrounded by surface components of peptides and phospholipids.

Before considering the role of the individual apoproteins in lipid metabolism it is appropriate to briefly describe the interconversions of the various lipoprotein classes during the catabolism of chylomicra and very low density lipoproteins, VLDL (Fig. 6.1).

Triglyceride-rich lipoproteins are synthesized and secreted from the small intestine and liver as chylomicra and VLDL. After circulation to peripheral tissues (muscle, adipose tissue and heart) they are delipidated by the action of lipolytic enzymes (such as lipoprotein lipase and hepatic lipase) to smaller particles (intermediate-density lipoproteins), which can undergo further catabolism to yield low-density lipoprotein (LDL) and chylomicra remnants. During the breakdown of triglyceride-rich lipoproteins in plasma, the C-apoproteins and some surface phospholipids are lost from the particle and may associate with high-density lipoproteins (HDL) for recycling onto newly formed VLDL. Low-density lipoprotein is degraded by the liver and peripheral tissues containing specific cell-surface receptors for the binding of LDL, endocytosis is stimulated and lysosomal breakdown of the particle occurs. This leads to the inhibition of the intracellular pathways of cholesterol biosynthesis by repression of 3-hydroxy-3-methylglutaryl co-enzyme-A reductase and an increase of intracellular esterification of cholesterol by an induction of another enzyme, a cholesteryl acyltransferase. High-density lipoprotein is mainly synthesized in the

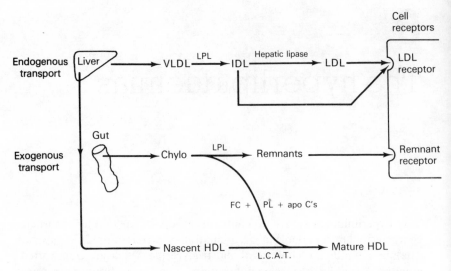

Fig. 6.1 Simplified scheme for lipid transport. Abbreviations: VLDL = very low density lipoprotein; IDL = intermediate density lipoprotein; LDL = low density lipoprotein; FC = free cholesterol; PL = phospholipids; apoC = C-apolipoproteins; LPL = lipoprotein lipase; LCAT = lecithin cholesteryl acyltransferase and HDL = high density lipoprotein.

intestine and liver. The HDL of hepatic origin contains predominantly E-apoprotein, whereas HDL of intestinal origin contains mainly A-apoprotein. There are at least two major classes of mature HDL particles, HDL_2 and HDL_3, of overall diameter 9.5–10nm and 7.0–7.5nm, respectively. It is possible that during the breakdown of VLDL to LDL some surface components (peptides and phospholipids) associate with HDL_3, converting it into a particle resembling HDL_2. It is thus apparent that there is a complex interconversion of these particles during transport of lipid between tissues.

The apolipoproteins
There are at least eight different apoproteins distributed throughout the lipoprotein system. The amino acid sequences of six of them have already been determined. The apoproteins were initially considered to serve a structural role in the formation and stabilization of the lipoprotein particle. However, it is now realized that many of them (e.g. Apo A-1, apo-B, apo C-II, apo C-III and apo-E) may have a functional role regulating enzymes or interacting with receptors involved in the catabolic pathways of lipoproteins in peripheral tissues. A summary of these particles and peptides is presented in Tables 6.1 and 6.2.

Table 6.1 Composition and properties of the human plasma lipoproteins

Properties	Chylomicrons	VLDL	LDL	HDL
Density (hydrated)	<0.95	0.95–1.006	1.006–1.063	1.063–1.210
Electrophoretic mobility	Origin	pre-beta	beta	alpha
Major apoproteins (% total):				
Apo AI	7.4	trace	–	67
Apo AII	4.2	trace	–	22
Apo B	22.5	36.9	98	trace
Apo CI	15	3.3	trace	1–3
Apo CII	15	6.7	trace	1–3
Apo CIII	36	40	trace	3–5
Apo E	–	13	trace	–
Lipid composition (%)				
Triglyceride	85	55	7	5
Cholesterol	. 6	17	50	35
Phospholipid	9	28	43	60

Table 6.2 The properties of human apolipoproteins. Abbreviations: LDL = low density lipoprotein; LCAT = lecithin cholesteryl acyl transferase and LPL = lipoprotein lipase

Apoproteins	Molecular weight	Number of amino acids	Site of synthesis	Function
A-I	28 300	243	Intestine/liver	Activates LCAT
A-II	17 000	154	Intestine/liver	–
B-100	549 000	–	Liver	⎧ Binds to LDL receptor +
B-48	246 000	–	Intestine	⎨ Triglyceride transport
C-I	6 331	57	Liver	Activates LCAT
C-II	8 837	78	Liver	Activates LPL
C-III	8 764	79	Liver	? inhibits LPL
E	33 000	299	Liver/intestine macrophage	?binds to liver receptor

Classification of the hyperlipidaemias

These disorders can be classified on the basis of which specific class of lipoprotein accumulates in plasma. The classification of the hyperlipidaemias on the basis of abnormalities of apolipoproteins, including the absence or primary structural defects in specific apolipoproteins, is potentially very useful. It also provides a rationale for the application of particular lipoprotein genes in the study of the aetiology of some of these disorders.

The diagnosis of a hyperlipidaemia rests upon identification of the elevated plasma lipid and the lipoprotein(s) on which it is transported. After discovery of a particular hyperlipidaemia it is useful to further characterize the lipid disorder as:

1. primary –differentiated into monogenic, polygenic forms, or non-inherited forms, or

2. secondary to systemic disease, nutrition or life-style habits, (e.g. alcohol excess).

Laboratory analysis of the lipids and lipoproteins provides the method for distinguishing the five major hyperlipoproteinaemias. Each type is defined by a pattern of lipoprotein accumulation and is not a homogenous entity from a clinical, genetic or pathophysiological viewpoint.

Type I hyperlipidaemia

Type I is defined by the presence of fasting hyperchylomicronaemia, with the subject on a 'normal' diet. When fat intake is restricted to less than 20g/day, the chylomicrons are gradually reduced in concentration and may disappear. Patients with this disease have a history of fatty food intolerance and may have recurrent bouts of pancreatitis. Two major molecular defects have now been identified in this disease. The classic defect is a deficiency of the enzyme lipoprotein lipase, specifically the extrahepatic lipoprotein lipase. A second defect due to the absence of the co-factor for lipoprotein lipase, apoprotein C-II, has also been identified as a cause of Type I hyperlipoproteinaemia. Although Type 1 is usually familial (inherited as an autosomal recessive), the lipoprotein pattern may be produced secondary to other systemic disorders such as systemic lupus erythematosis, the macroglobulinaemias and occasionally diabetic ketoacidosis.

The distinction between primary and secondary Type I hyper-lipidaemia is usually easily made. The familial form usually presents in childhood, with hepatosplenomegaly, eruptive xanthomas and lipaemia retinalis. Recurrent pancreatitis is the main clinical problem and despite very high levels of chylomicron-triglycerides, there is little evidence for an increased incidence of premature vascular disease.

Type II hyperlipidaemia

Type II hyperlipidaemias are subdivided into IIa and IIb lipoprotein patterns. The Type IIa lipoprotein pattern is characterized by increased

LDL with normal VLDL. Plasma cholesterol is elevated, triglycerides are normal and the plasma is clear.

Type IIb is characterized by increased LDL-cholesterol as well as an increase in VLDL-cholesterol and triglyceride. Plasma triglycerides are moderately elevated, in the absence of a floating intermediate-density lipoprotein (IDL). Occasionally it is necessary to perform an ultra-centrifugal study to differentiate Types IIb from III.

Three major genetic types of hypercholesterolaemia are associated with Type II hyperlipoproteinaemia. These include familial hypercholesterolaemia (FH) and familial combined hyperlipoproteinaemia (FCH), both of which are inherited as autosomal dominant disorders, and a hypercholesterolaemia of variable phenotype which is not inherited in a simple Mendelian fashion. However, there is strong familial clustering in the distribution of the latter hypercholesterolaemia in kindreds, and this may be based on a polygenic form of inheritance, with two or more defective genes required before the disease is expressed.

Acquired Type II hyperlipoproteinaemia is often observed as a result of excessive intake of cholesterol and saturated fats in the diet and is wide-spread in western industrialized countries. It is presumed to be one of the many reasons for the high prevalence of atherosclerosis in these areas. However, genetic mechanisms may well play an important aetiological role in these acquired forms of hypercholesterolaemia. Many individuals are resistant to the hypercholesterolaemic effects of a high cholesterol diet. Others become hypercholesterolaemic even with moderate loading of dietary fat and are particularly susceptible to such consequences as atherosclerosis. This variable susceptibility to environmental stresses may well have a genetic basis. Other causes of acquired hyperlipoproteinaemia Type II, such as hypothyroidism, the nephrotic syndrome and the dysgammaglobulinaemias, must also be considered.

The most extensively studied of the hypercholesterolaemias is the familial form (familial hypercholesterolaemia). This has been shown in some cases to be due to a functional defect in the LDL receptor. This defect has now been demonstrated in many cell types, including liver, skin fibroblasts and fresh leucocytes, and is associated with defective catabolism of LDL *in vivo*. The molecular defects in familial combined hyperlipidaemia, or in the polygenic forms, are as yet unknown.

Type III hyperlipidaemia

This disorder is characterized by hypercholesterolaemia and hypertriglyceridaemia carried on an abnormal particle of intermediate density between VLDL and LDL, called IDL (or intermediate-density lipoprotein). This abnormal lipoprotein can be demonstrated as a broad beta band on cellulose acetate electrophoresis. For accurate diagnosis an ultracentrifugal study is required to demonstrate the presence of floating beta (or IDL) lipoprotein and an analysis of the E-apoprotein isoforms. The metabolic defect in Type III hyperlipidaemia has been shown to be a defect in chylomicron remnant removal. This defeçt is often associated with the presence of a particular apoprotein E polymorphic variant. The E-apoproteins exist as three major polymorphic variants designated as E_2, E_3 and E_4 and characterized by differing isoelectric focussing patterns. The biochemical basis for the difference in charge of the apo E variants is due to cysteine/arginine substitutions at three different residues in the peptide. The major variants found in patients with Type III hyperlipidaemia are E_2/E_2 where cysteine residues are found at each of these sites.

This particular apo E variant may be functionally defective, perhaps resulting in impaired catabolism of the chylomicron remnant and the accumulation of IDL. However, a number of studies suggest that the presence of the E_2/E_2 phenotype is not in itself sufficient for the development of the Type III disorder. Coexisting genetic defects (e.g. diabetes mellitus) or environmental factors (such as obesity or hypothyroidism) may be important for the occurrence of the disease.

Type IV hyperlipidaemia
Type IV hyperlipoproteinaemia is characterized by elevations of plasma triglycerides and VLDL, and is often secondary to a wide variety of diseases and dietary habits. Furthermore, several different genetic forms may express as a Type IV phenotype, including familial combined hyperlipidaemia (FCH) and familial hypertriglyceridaemia. Since there are many ways of acquiring the Type IV phenotype, clinical assessment should include a careful distinction between primary and secondary causes. Furthermore, since triglycerides may fall abruptly during calorie restriction and weight reduction, it is particularly important to obtain fasting blood for measurement of triglyceride levels when the patient is on his habitual diet and the weight is stable. The commonly encountered causes of secondary Type IV hyperlipoproteinaemia include diabetes mellitus, excessive alcohol intake, hypothyroidism, renal disease and exogenous oestrogen therapy.

Clinical examination is not particularly useful in discriminating between primary and secondary hypertriglyceridaemia. Eruptive xanthomas may occur in about 15 per cent of patients with Type IV, but only when the triglycerides are markedly elevated. Systemic disorders also modify the occurrence of an underlying primary hypertriglyceridaemia. A good example is the increased severity of familial hypertriglyceridaemia in the presence of poorly controlled diabetes mellitus. The severe alcoholic lipaemias and those produced by exogenous oestrogen therapy also seem to occur in patients with underlying lipid intolerance.

Studies of the pathophysiology of Type IV hyperlipidaemia have implicated an increased VLDL production rate by the liver and/or a defective VLDL clearance from the plasma. However, the precise molecular defects are as yet unknown, and it is probable that the Type IV phenotype includes several different genetic variants. In addition, the expression of the disorder is markedly influenced by environmental factors.

Type V hyperlipidaemia

Type V hyperlipoproteinaemia is characterized by elevated plasma triglycerides due to both increased VLDL and chylomicrons. Plasma cholesterol may be marginally or moderately increased and HDL –cholesterol is usually normal or low. The plasma is usually opaque and a floating creamy layer above the turbid plasma may be observed. Patients with the Type V phenotype have considerably higher triglyceride levels than patients with Type IV, but major difficulties may arise in distinguishing Type V from Type IV, as the Type V pattern is often transient. Many subjects with Type V hyperlipidaemia reduce their chylomicron levels even with moderate reduction in dietary triglyceride.

As with Type IV, Type V hyperlipidaemia is often secondary to a wide variety of diseases and life-styles. The list is broadly similar to that

Table 6.3 A summary of the primary hyperlipidaemias

WHO type	Lipoprotein changes	Causes
I	Chylos increased, HDL and LDL reduced	Lipoprotein lipase deficiency, Apo-CII deficiency
IIa	LDL increased	Familial hypercholesterolaemia, Polygenic hypercholesterolaemia
IIb	LDL and VLDL increased, HDL may be low	Familial combined hyperlipidaemia
III	IDL (chylo remnants) increased, LDL and HDL low	Associated with gene polymorphism of Apo E
IV	VLDL increased, HDL low	Familial hypertriglyceridaemia, Familial combined hyperlipidaemia, Polygenic hyperlipidaemia
V	VLDL, chylos increased HDL low	Familial hypertriglyceridaemia, Lipoprotein lipase deficiency

outlined for Type IV. Consequently, a careful history is needed to establish whether the disorder is primary or secondary.

Familial Type V hyperlipidaemia is often associated with a history of recurrent abdominal pain due to pancreatitis, hepatosplenomegaly, eruptive xanthomas and lipaemia retinalis. More than 75 per cent of such patients will have impaired glucose tolerance.

The chylomicronaemia of Type V (similar qualitatively to Type I) suggests that Type V might represent a partial defect in the peripheral lipolytic mechanisms, resulting in delayed clearance of chylomicrons and VLDL. However, as is the case with type IV, a number of different molecular mechanisms are probably implicated in the pathogenesis, which still remain to be characterized. A summary of the salient features of the hyperlipidaemias is presented in Table 6.3.

Clinical consequence of the hyperlipidaemias

Clinical observations have suggested for many years a central role for the lipoproteins in the aetiology of coronary heart disease and premature atherosclerosis. The lifelong elevation of LDL concentrations in familial hypercholesterolaemia is associated with a several-fold excess risk of premature coronary heart disease. In subjects who are homozygous for familial hypercholesterolaemia, clinical symptoms such as aortic stenosis secondary to atheromatous deposits on the aortic ring, and ischaemic cardiac pain can present in early childhood. Death due to severe atherosclerosis before the age of 20 years is usual in the untreated homozygote. Concentrations of LDL-cholesterol are directly related and predict the risk of coronary heart disease over a wide age range. High-density lipoprotein concentrations are also strongly predictive for the risk of coronary heart disease, the relationship being inverse. Coronary heart disease has been reported to be rare in a familial syndrome characterized by high HDL and low LDL concentrations. These associations have prompted extensive research into the mechanisms whereby the lipoproteins may influence the atherosclerotic process.

Although there is very strong epidemiological and experimental evidence for the atherogenic properties of LDL, the atherogenicity of the triglyceride-rich lipoproteins is unclear. Very low-density lipoprotein carries a relatively small amount of cholesterol and since it is a relatively large particle (compared to LDL) it poorly penetrates the intima of the arterial wall. However, in epidemiological studies hypertriglyceridaemia has been found to associate with both premature coronary heart disease and peripheral vascular disease. It is not clear whether this association implies a direct causal relationship between the two or is secondary to a disturbance of the other lipoproteins.

In summary, the hyperlipidaemias are a heterogeneous group of disorders ranging in frequency from rare to common in western populations, and strongly implicated in the aetiology of premature atherosclerosis. Some have a definite genetic abnormality whilst others depend on a complex interaction between ill-defined genetic factors and environmental factors before full manifestation of the disease. A specific genetic diagnosis however should be established whenever possible. This may help in the understanding of the aetiology of these disorders, as well as alerting the clinician to survey the family in order to identify relatives at risk who may require treatment. A summary of well-defined monogenic hyperlipidaemias is given in Table 6.4. In six of these

Table 6.4 A genetic classification of the hyperlipidaemias

Disorder	Estimated prevalence
Monogenic	
1. Apolipoprotein mutations	
Familial apo C-II deficiency	$<1 : 1\ 000\ 000$
Apoprotein A-I mutations	$1 : 1\ 000\ 000$
Familial type III (apoprotein (E_2/E_2)	$1 : 10\text{-}100\ 000$
2. Receptor mutations	
αFamilial hypercholesterolaemia	$1 : 500$
3. Enzyme mutations	
Familial lipoprotein lipase deficiency	$<1 : 100\ 000$
Familial LCAT deficiency	$<1 : 1\ 000\ 000$
Ill defined, possibly polygenic disorders	
Familial hypertriglyceridaemia	$1 : 500$
Familial polygenic hypercholesterolaemia	?
Familial combined hyperlipidaemia	$1 : 300$

disorders the molecular defect is established and the prevalence of the disorders can be estimated. The prevalence of the polygenic or poorly defined primary hyperlipidaemias is more difficult to estimate because the distribution of the lipoprotein concentrations in the population at large is continuous and thus diagnosis depends on the assignment of arbitrary cut off points.

It is in the study of these poorly understood polygenic disorders that the application of recombinant DNA technology may hold such promise, by identifying genes that contribute to the phenotype. Some of the apolipoprotein genes are now available for investigating the aetiology of the polygenic hyperlipidaemias and are considered in detail below.

The apolipoprotein genes

It has been established that there are at least eight different apolipoproteins and the amino acid sequences of six of these peptides have been elucidated. Using a synthetic oligonucleotide as a probe, cDNA clones coding for five of these peptides have been identified and characterized. By selecting a favourable region of the known amino acid sequence, i.e. a sequence of amino acids which has a low degeneracy in the genetic code, specific oligonucleotides (usually 15 or 17 nucleotides in length) are constructed and can be used as probes to screen an adult human cDNA liver library. Clones hybridizing with the labelled oligonucleotide probe can then be characterized and sequenced, and the cDNA clones coding for the appropriate apolipoprotein may be identified. This approach requires knowledge of the primary amino acid sequence as well as suitable abundance of mRNA in the tissue source of the cDNA library ('high' abundance being defined as greater than one per cent of the total mRNA). Fortunately, the level of mRNA encoding the apolipoproteins is usually in excess of the minimum required, and this approach has been successful in isolating cDNA clones coding for apo A-1, apo A-II, apo C-II, apo C-III and apo E. A brief description of the molecular and functional properties of these peptides has been presented in Table 6.2 (p.85). Of interest is the possibility that some of the lipoprotein genes arose by duplication from a common ancestral gene several million years ago. It is also of interest that at least two types of polymorphisms have arisen in the apolipoprotein system. There is an amino acid polymorphism exemplified by the E-apoprotein variants differing at two main sites (112 and 158) in the peptide producing three common variants – E_2, E_3 and E_4.

Then there is a post-translational variation, best exemplified in apo C-III (a single chain peptide of 79 residues and molecular weight of 8764 daltons). This peptide can occur in three isomorphic forms depending on the number of sialic acid residues attached to threonine 74. Apo C-III-0, apo C-III-1 and apo C-III-2 contain zero, one or two moles of sialic acid per mole of peptide respectively and give rise to quite different mobilities on isoelectric focussing. It is possible that these polymorphic variants subserve slightly different functional roles in the process of lipid transport amongst tissues, since variation in their percentage proportions can be associated with a hyperlipidaemia.

The use of the human apolipoprotein gene probes in the study of genetic disorders of lipoprotein metabolism is still in its infancy. Hitherto, the approach has been to identify and characterize abnormalities of protein structure and function in individuals with a clearly defined hyperlipidaemia. Now the approach can be extended.

Using these gene specific probes it is hoped to gain a deeper insight into the genetic determinants of the various hyperlipidaemias in several ways:

1. they will provide information as to whether the gene has undergone structural rearrangements;

2. if the gene is present mRNA/cDNA hybridization experiments will confirm whether the gene is transcribed; or

3. detection of differences in DNA sequence due to single base changes, deletions or insertions that are estimated to occur once in every 300 base pairs in the normal population.

These DNA variations may be detected as restriction fragment length polymorphisms (RFLPs) and are inherited in a simple Mendelian fashion. The majority of such DNA variations previously described have not been shown to be associated with any protein abnormalities or disease states. However, in some cases, the restriction site polymorphism shows population disequilibrium with a particular disease phenotype. One such example described on p.63 is a mutant Hpa1 site producing a restriction site polymorphism flanking the beta globin gene that segregates wth sickle cell disease in 80 per cent of a West African population. Using this approach it may be possible by extensive population studies to identify polymorphisms that segregate with some of the genetically determined hyperlipidaemias, without even knowing the identity of the abnormal gene or genes involved in the disease. If this were successful it may eventually be possible to predict the level of risk for an individual to develop one of the polygenic hyperlipidaemias in early postnatal life. The appropriate dietary and lifestyle changes could be instituted at an early age with the aim of delaying the onset of premature atherosclerosis.

Clinical studies with the apolipoprotein genes

The apolipoproteins A-I and C-III genes

The first reports of the application of cloned human apolipoprotein genes to the study of disease appeared simultaneously in the scientific literature in early 1983. Both reports describe the use of apo A-1 cDNA probes in the restriction enzyme analysis of human chromosomal DNA.

In one case two sisters were studied who exhibited an unique combination of clinical and biochemical abnormalities, including skin and tendon xanthomas, corneal clouding and severe premature coronary atherosclerosis associated with very low HDL levels and deficiencies of two apoproteins, namely apo A-1 and apo C-III. Restriction enzyme analysis using a cDNA apo A-1 probe revealed a restriction site polymorphism at the apo A-1 gene locus in these individuals, which was subsequently demonstrated to be due to at least 6.5 kb DNA insertion in the coding region of the apo A-1 gene. Both probands were demonstrated to be homozygous for this defect; and first degree relatives heterozygous for this locus were found to have intermediate levels of HDL, apo A-1 and apo C-III, but were asymptomatic and clinically unaffected.

Previous analysis of amino-acid sequence data has suggested that the genes for apo A-1 and apo C-III are derived by gene duplication from a common evolutionary precursor. In addition, it was noted that the 6.5 kb insert in the apo A-1 gene correlated with a deficiency of both apo A-1 and apo C-III in this particular family with premature atherosclerosis. It was, therefore, speculated that a close linkage may exist between the apo A-1 and apo C-III genes. To examine this possibility, a cDNA probe was isolated from a human liver cDNA library using a synthetically prepared oligonucleotide probe as previously described. A fully characterized genomic clone containing the entire apo A-1 gene was prepared, digested with various restriction endonucleases, and hybridized with the apo C-III gene probe. It was found that the large genomic apo A-1 clone contained DNA sequences strongly homologous to the apo C-III cDNA probe and further characterization and sequencing of the genomic sequences flanking the apo A-1 gene confirmed the presence of the gene coding for apolipoprotein C-III, situated approximately 2.6 kb downstream from

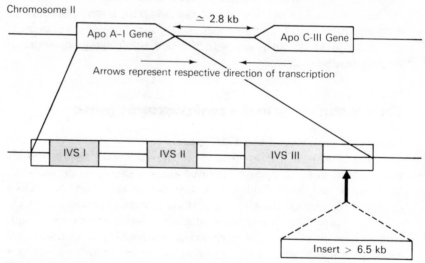

Fig. 6.2 The organization of the apoA-I/C-III gene complex in a patient with familial deficiency of both apolipoproteins A-I and C-III. In the probands with familial deficiency of both apolipoproteins A-I and C-III, a large insert of DNA is located in the coding region of the apoA-I gene. This insert is thought to consist of at least 6.5 kb.

the 3'-end of the apo A-1 gene. Furthermore, it appears that they are convergently transcribed as summarized in Fig. 6.2.

These results support the previous suggestion that the apo A-1 and apo C-III genes may be evolutionarily related. Furthermore, they indicate that these apolipoprotein genes may be co-ordinately regulated (or share common controls for gene expression) as suggested by two probands who exhibit complete absence of both apo A-1 and C-III proteins when they possess a 6.5 kb insert in the coding region of the A-1 gene. This apo A-1/C-III gene cluster has now been located by filter hybridization analysis of human-mouse cell hybrids to the long arm of chromosome 11. It is not yet clear how closely situated this gene cluster is to other genes such as insulin, beta-globin and lactate dehydrogenase on the short arm of chromosome 11 (Fig. 6.3).

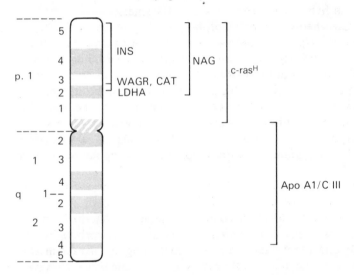

Fig. 6.3 A diagrammatic map of the human chromosome 11. Abbreviations used are: INS = insulin; CAT = catalase and c-ras^H = c-Harvey ras oncogene. This is a standard map of the banding pattern of one chromatid of chromosome 11 as seen at metaphase; more bands are observed at early prophase. All bands stain with reagents that appear to be specific for A-T rich DNA sequences.

In another study, using a different cDNA probe for apo A-1 and restricting human genomic DNA with Sst I endonuclease, a restriction fragment length polymorphism in the 3'-flanking region of the apo A-1 gene has been identified in approximately five per cent of a healthy population, but is found in some 35 per cent of hypertriglyceridaemic patients exhibiting a lipoprotein phenotype IV or V (Table 6.3, p.89). Homozygosity for these alleles does not result in increased severity of the hypertriglyceridaemia. Furthermore, hypertriglyceridaemic patients possessing the polymorphism do not appear to have significantly altered concentrations of apolipoprotein A-1 or HDL, nor do they have differing distributions of the apo C-III isoforms when compared to hypertriglyceridaemic patients possessing the common A-1 alleles.

Further gene mapping suggested that this restriction fragment length polymorphism related to the apo A-1 gene is not caused by any extensive deletion or insertion in the 3′-flanking region, but may be caused by a cytosine to guanine transversional mutation, thus creating a new Sst I cleavage site by producing the appropriate recognition sequence GAGCTC. This polymorphic locus has subsequently been located to the 3′ non-coding region of the closely linked apo C-III gene. This observation is confirmed by restriction enzyme analysis of these individuals and hybridizing with the apo C-III gene.

It is not clear whether this polymorphism directly relates to the hyper-triglyceridaemia, especially as the hypertriglyceridaemic population studied represents a fairly diverse and heterogenous group. Furthermore, a significant racial variation of this polymorphism is observed, with a high prevalence of the polymorphic allele being found in normolipaemic Chinese and Japanese subjects. One explanation may be that this polymorphism is in linkage disequilibrium with genetic factors that might predispose an individual to hyperlipidaemia in a Caucasian population, but is randomly distributed amongst the population in other racial groups.

Restriction mapping of the A-1 locus has also been performed on individuals with Tangier disease and fish eye disease. Both are distinct monogenic disorders of lipoprotein metabolism inherited in an autosomal recessive manner. Both disorders are characterized by low levels of HDL and apo A-1 concentrations suggesting that in each disease there may be a genetic defect at the apo A-1/C-III gene locus. However, restriction enzyme analysis reveals no such gross alteration of DNA organization as found in the apo A-1/CIII deficiency syndrome. However, small deletions (of less than 500 base pairs) or point mutations which may affect either gene expression or the primary structure of apo A-1 may not necessarily be revealed by this approach and may require the sequencing of the gene in affected individuals for a complete assessment.

Apolipoprotein ε gene

As yet, no restriction length fragment polymorphisms suitable for population or linkage studies in pedigrees have been demonstrated around the apo ε gene locus. However, DNA sequence analysis has demonstrated that the cysteine/arginine substitution which occur within apo E molecule at position 112 and 158 to produce the various apo E polymorphic variants may result from a single base substitution in the first position at each of these codons. This supports the hypothesis that the apo E protein polymorphisms are due to DNA mutations in the coding region of the apo Ɛ gene, which in turn may contribute to the phenotypic expression of Type III hyperlipoproteinaemia.

Apolipoprotein C-II gene
A cDNA clone for human apolipoprotein C-II has been used to detect a common polymorphism using the restriction endonuclease Taq I. This polymorphism is probably caused by a single base change approximately 2 kb from the 3′-end of the gene. The polymorphism may be used to define two alleles of the apo C-II gene, but the frequency of the two alleles is not significantly different in patient groups with various types of hyperlipidaemias compared to control subjects. It thus appears that the Taq I polymorphism of the apo C-II gene is not in linkage disequilibrium with genetic factors that might predispose an individual to hyperlipidaemia. It may, therefore, be an example of a neutral polymorphism, which is expected to be more typical of the majority of restriction fragment polymorphisms so far reported (for example within the globin gene cluster). This, however, does not in any way exclude the possibility of the apo C-II gene being an important component in predisposing individuals to develop hypertriglyceridaemia.

The application of recombinant DNA technology and the study of the apolipoprotein genes in the aetiology of hyperlipidaemia have identified four different categories of DNA polymorphisms, namely:

1. Insertion of a DNA sequence, resulting in altered expression of two closely linked genes, the apo A-1 and apo C-III genes, with severe clinical consequences.

2. Linked polymorphism, in this case a point mutation, which may be in linkage disequilibrium with other gene(s) that may confer susceptibility to hyperlipidaemia.

3. Intragenic point mutations giving rise to protein variants (e.g. the apo E_2 isoform) which may be partly responsible for expression of the Type III phenotype.

4. Neutral polymorphism which appears to be unrelated to any hyperlipidaemic phenotype.

These constitute good examples of all the types of polymorphic variants that are likely to be encountered in such studies.

Future prospects

The methodology and concepts which have been developed in the study of haemoglobinopathies may be applied directly to the study of the apolipoproteins and lipid transport. The conceptual framework for the extension of this method of analysis has been outlined and the only limitation to the wider application of DNA analysis to the hyper-lipidaemias is the number of human gene probes that have been isolated and which show significant involvement in the hyperlipidaemias. However, this should not be a limiting factor for very much longer, as the number of genes being isolated and characterized are increasing rapidly. From a theoretical viewpoint, it is anticipated that great interest will focus on the application of gene probes specifying such proteins as the LDL receptor, lipoprotein lipase and the B apolipoprotein.

Ultimately, it is in the application of multiple gene analysis in the families of patients with polygenic hyperlipidaemia that most information will be gained. It may be that different combinations of DNA polymorphisms result in the expression of diverse hyperlipidaemic phenotypes; and family studies may provide linkage data to clarify this point.

In addition, speculation based on amino acid sequence data suggests that the apolipoproteins A-1, A-II, C-I and C-III are all derived from a common ancestral precursor. The A-1 and C-III genes have already been shown to be closely linked and sequence analysis of the apo A-1 gene suggests that its structure may be composed of tandemly repeated DNA sequences which have a significant degree of homology. This observation suggests that intragenic recombination may have been responsible for the apo A-1 gene expansion. Isolation and characterization of the other apolipoprotein genes, and comparison of their structure with the apo A-1 gene, may well clarify the evolutionary relationships, if any, amongst these genes.

For the future, there is very little doubt that the hyperlipoprotein-aemias and atherosclerosis will provide a fertile field of study, particularly with recombinant DNA technology providing apolipo-protein gene probes as investigative tools. The role of genetic factors in determining the plasma levels of VLDL, LDL and HDL may ultimately provide a better understanding of the variability of plasma lipids between individuals and may also help to explain their differing predisposition to atherosclerosis. Rapid expansion in the understanding of this area of polygenic disease is imminent.

Further reading

Havel, J.R. ed. (1982). *Lipid Disorders. Medical Clinics of North America*, Vol. 66, No. 2. W.B. Saunders and Co., Philadelphia. (Many chapters by different authors on all aspects of lipid disorders.)

Lewis, B. (1976). *The Hyperlipidaemias: Clinical and Laboratory Practice*. Blackwell Scientific Publications, Oxford.
(A good general text introducing the hyperlipidaemias.)
Myant, N.B. (1982). *Biology of Cholesterol*. Heinemann Medical, London.
(A comprehensive specialist monograph.)
Rifkind, B.M. and Levy, R.I. (1977). *Hyperlipidaemias: Diagnosis and Therapy*. Grune and Stratton, New York.
(A good multi-author account of the hyperlipidaemias.)

7

Diabetes mellitus:

Pathophysiology

Diabetes mellitus is a heterogeneous disease associated variably with:
1. chronic elevation of blood glucose,
2. loss of glucose in the urine, and
3. an excessive mobilization of fat from adipose tissue, which in extreme cases leads to a ketoacidosis.

It is a common disorder occurring in more than two per cent of the UK population.

Diabetes can be usefully classified into two types: a disorder requiring insulin therapy (or insulin-dependent diabetes, IDDM, or Type I diabetes); and a type not requiring insulin therapy (or non-insulin dependent diabetes, NIDDM, or Type II diabetes). For convenience, the Type I and II classification will be used. There are numerous secondary causes of the diabetic syndrome and a fuller classification is presented in Table 7.1. In addition to diabetes mellitus, the term 'impaired glucose tolerance' is used to define a group of borderline diabetics who may not run the risk of developing typical diabetic complications but may still have twice the incidence of coronary heart disease.

Although precise diagnostic criteria have been laid down (World

Table 7.1 Classification of diabetic disorders

Primary diabetes mellitus;
      Type I : Insulin dependent
      Type II: Non insulin dependent
            Maturity onset diabetes of the young (MODY)
      Impaired glucose tolerance

Secondary diabetes mellitus;
      Gestational diabetes
      Hormonal imbalance (Cushing's disease, acromegaly)
      Drug induced
      Pancreatic disease (e.g. haemochromatosis)

Health Organization 1980) based on arbitrary levels of blood glucose reached after an oral glucose load, clinically the diagnosis is often not difficult to establish. Polyuria, polydipsia, weight loss and marked postprandial (or fasting) hyperglycaemia are usually sufficient to make a diagnosis.

Diabetes mellitus is a heterogeneous group of disorders and only in rare instances is the complete pathophysiology understood. For example, pancreatic destruction by neoplasm or infiltration (by amyloid or in haemochromatosis) may lead to insulin-dependent (or Type I) diabetes; but it is probable that more than 80 per cent of the islet cell mass needs to be destroyed before this occurs.

For the more usual types of diabetes a mixture of genetic and environmental factors may be involved, but the relative contribution and importance of each component needs clarification. Some aetiological factors that have been implicated for both Types I and II diabetes can be considered.

Genetics

It is well recognized that diabetes runs in families; but its mode of inheritance has so far defied analysis. Possibilities of a single gene defect with variable penetrance, or polygenic inheritance have been proposed. The disease is unlikely to be genetically homogeneous, and the genetic components may only lead to a predisposition or susceptibility to the disease when appropriate environmental factors are encountered, rather than directly determine the onset of the disease.

1. Twin studies

A study of twins at King's College Hospital London has shown that about 90 per cent of identical twins are concordant for Type II diabetes, whereas only 50 per cent are concordant for Type I diabetes. This striking difference in concordance emphasizes some of the possible genetic differences between these two disorders, and is supported by HLA distribution and family histories.

2. Family studies

The type of diabetes within a diabetic pedigree does not always breed 'true'. Thus of Type II probands 20 per cent may have affected siblings with the same form of diabetes and two per cent with Type I diabetes. This suggests multiple gene inheritance, with varying combinations producing either Type I or II diabetes.

3. Rare genetic syndromes

Glucose intolerance of clinical diabetes have been found to accompany

Table 7.2 A partial list of genetic syndromes associated with glucose intolerance

---

Inherited endocrine disorders
    Isolated growth hormone deficiency
    Hereditary panhypopituiary dwarfism
    Phaeochromocytoma
    Multiple endocrine adenomatosis

Inborn errors of metabolism
    Glycogen storage disease Type I
    Acute intermittent porphyria
    Hyperlipidaemias Type IV/V

Syndromes associated with pancreatic degeneration
    Hereditary relapsing pancreatitis
    Cystic fibrosis
    Haemochromatosis
    Alpha 1-antitrypsin deficiency

Syndromes associated with insulin resistance
    Myotonic dystrophy
    Lipoatrophic diabetes
    Acanthosis nigricans (with insulin resistance)

Miscellaneous disorders
    Huntington's chorea
    Friedrich's ataxia
    Lawrence-Moon-Biedl syndrome
    Down's syndrome
    Kleinfelters syndrome
    Turner's syndrome

---

over 40 distinct genetic syndromes. Some of these are listed in Table 7.2. This observation suggests that mutations at many different loci may associate with glucose intolerance. However, there are several rare insulin gene defects that produce a mutant insulin (see p. 108) which may have less biological activity than native insulin, and consequently is required in excess to maintain normal glucose homeostasis. This can lead to a clinical picture of Type II diabetes if additional environmental factors occur to increase peripheral resistance (such as obesity); otherwise the overproduction of a biologically less active insulin may never be discovered in adult life.

4. The HLA system

The short arm of chromosome 6 contains the HLA genes which code for antigens of the major histocompatibility system. HLA genes A, B and C code for surface glycoproteins found on nearly all nucleated cells. HLA D and the D-related locus (DR) code for surface antigens found predominantly on B lymphocytes and macrophages.

This region of chromosome 6 is highly polymorphic, having many different possible alleles at each locus (probably greater than 3×10^7 different combinations). The loci are very close together (0.15 centimorgans) and so there is very little recombination (i.e. crossovers at meiosis), and the various combinations of the HLA genes are transmitted to the next generation *en bloc* in 98 per cent of cases. This may, in part, explain certain combinations being in linkage disequilibrium, e.g. A1 and B8; A3 and B7; and for the preferential distribution of certain allelic combinations in different racial groups.

The recently described association of the DR antigens with Type I diabetes is particularly striking, conferring a 'risk' of 14 times the general population if an individual possesses both DR3 and DR4 antigens. Some 90 per cent of all newly diagnosed children with Type I diabetes have either DR3, DR4 or both antigens. However, whilst family studies show that siblings with Type I diabetes usually have the same HLA genotype, it does not explain why unaffected members of the same family may also have the same 'diabetogenic' HLA combinations. Perhaps other genes outside the HLA system are required to confer susceptibility; or possession of particular HLA genes may affect immune responsiveness to various environmental factors (such as viruses) which may favour destruction of the pancreatic islets.

The HLA system influences the immune status of an individual and there is a well-recognized association between diabetes and other organ specific immune disorders such as hypothyroidism or Addison's disease. In these particular disorders, thyroid and adrenal antibodies can be present long before diagnosis; and this may be the same for Type I diabetes and the presence of circulating islet cell antibodies. Two major islet cell antibodies can be detected: a surface antibody that does not fix complement, and a microsomal antibody of which a fraction is complement-fixing. There is no evidence as yet that these autoantibodies are pathogenic for the development of diabetes mellitus *in vivo*; and they may occur secondarily to islet cell damage. However, they may be of prognostic significance in unaffected individuals for the future onset of diabetes mellitus.

Finally the genetic heterogeneity of diabetes is supported by HLA studies since no association has been found relating to Type II diabetes, suggesting that Type I and II diabetes may have separate genetic determinants.

Environmental factors

It is likely that certain environmental factors are required to precipitate the onset of both Type I and Type II diabetes. In the former, viruses have been frequently implicated, including mumps, Coxsackie B, rubella and the Epstein-Barr virus. In the latter nutritional factors, particularly the presence of obesity may lead to peripheral resistance to the action of insulin.

Obesity may reduce the number or impair the affinity of insulin receptors in such organs as adipose tissue or muscle, and lead to hyperinsulinaemia. The pancreatic B-cells may be able to compensate for this peripheral resistance up to a point by increasing the output of insulin. However, pancreatic insufficiency may develop and when the secretion of insulin for the prevailing state of insulin resistance becomes inadequate Type II diabetes may result. This can be aggravated by the excess secretion of counter-regulatory hormones to insulin, such as corticosteroids (as in Cushing's disease) or growth hormone (as in acromegaly).

The insulin gene and diabetes-related disorders

Recent advances in recombinant DNA methods now permit a direct analysis of the insulin gene and other genes that may contribute to the genetics of diabetes and its related disorders. The majority of this work has been performed with the insulin gene, but extensions to the insulin-receptor gene and HLA genes are in progress. The rest of this chapter will describe current studies related to the insulin gene. The gene was first isolated, cloned and sequenced by G.I. Bell in 1980. Messenger RNA was extracted from a human insulinoma (a large proportion of which codes for insulin); and then using a rat cDNA gene probe he isolated mRNA for human insulin, and hence obtained a cDNA clone for the hormone using reverse transcriptase (Fig. 4.3, p.49). The latter clone was then used as a probe to isolate the human insulin gene from a genomic library.

Insulin gene structure

The human insulin gene, located on the short arm of chromosome 11, is 1355 base pairs in length, comprising three coding regions (or exons) separated by two introns (Fig. 7.1). The first exon contains DNA sequences specifying ribosomal binding sites on the final mRNA product. Within the second exon is the start codon (ATG) followed by sequences coding for the signal peptide, B chain and C peptide. The DNA sequence coding the C peptide is interrupted by a second intron. The sequence for the A chain is found in the third exon. At the 3′-end of the gene the site of the polyadenine (poly A) tail is located 74 nucleotides from the stop codon.

Regulatory sequences are found in the 5′-flanking region. The promotor region (or TATAA sequence) which binds RNA polymerase is

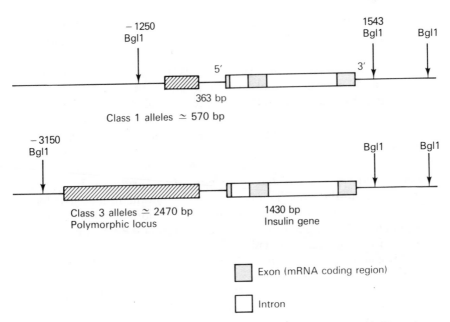

Fig. 7.1 A map of the human insulin gene located on chromosome 11. Note the large insertions (hatched areas) at the 5′-end of the gene.

located 25 base pairs from exon 1; and a gene enhancer sequence may occur between bases 168–258 from exon 1.

The first product of the insulin gene, or its primary transcript, contains all the transcribed sequence from the first nucleotide of exon 1 to the site of the poly-A tail on the 3′-side of the gene, including the introns. The next step involves enzymatic splicing out of the two introns, leaving the mature mRNA. Subsequently, the mRNA is translated into the peptide product of the insulin gene, pre-proinsulin, and is available for storage and secretion.

DNA variation in and around the insulin gene

Within the coding sequence

Insulin is one of the most closely conserved biological molecules in nature and this is reflected in the conservation of the amino-acid sequence in phylogenetically older species. For example, hagfish insulin has 80 per cent homology with human insulin. At the DNA level only a few mammals have been shown have a different gene structure. Rat, mouse and several fish species have been shown to possess two separate non-allelic insulin genes. The rat insulin gene 1 differs from gene 2 by not having the first intron. Rat insulin gene 2 is almost identical in DNA sequence to the human insulin gene, possessing three exons and two introns.

Within the human insulin gene there is a certain amount of allelic variation. Of four genes that have been sequenced, they differed from each other by four nucleotides. The positions of these polymorphisms were one within intron 1; one within intron 2; and two in the 3'-untranslated region. They appeared to be without pathological effects.

DNA insertions in the 5'-flanking region of the insulin gene

In contrast to the close homology found within the insulin gene locus amongst animal species, there is a highly polymorphic region of DNA beginning 363 base pairs from the start of insulin mRNA synthesis (the hatched box of Fig. 7.1). This region can be broadly subdivided into alleles containing one of three DNA inserts of variable length: short DNA insertions, 0–600 base pairs (Class 1 allelle); intermediate sized insertions, 600–1600 base pairs (Class 2 allele); and long DNA insertions of 1600–2200 base pairs (Class 3 allele). The nucleotide structure of these three insertions are very similar being composed of a variable number of a 14 base pair oligonucleotide of consensus sequence, ACAGGGGTGT-GGGG.

Hence the Class 1, 2 and 3 alleles differ only in possessing on average 40, 80 or 160 tandem duplications of this oligonucleotide, respectively. Although it is likely from nucleotide sequence data that nearly every individual may have slight differences in the total nucleotide sequence of the insertion class, for the purpose of clinical studies, it is still not possible to make use of this information. For such studies restriction enzyme analysis is used, which even in the most capable hands can only detect differences of 50 base pairs in length between allelic variants. Man, being diploid, inherits an insulin gene allele from both parents and hence the following genotypes can be observed: 1/1 (homozygous small); 1/2, 1/3 (heterozygous for large and small); and 2/2, 2/3 and 3/3 (homozygous large). This region can therefore be used as a genetic marker for the two parental insulin genes as more than 63 per cent of individuals are heterozygous with respect to length at this point. In practice, in Caucasian subjects the Class 2 allele is uncommon and for this reason most studies have combined data of the Class 2 with the Class 3 allele. The bimodal distribution of DNA inserts in Caucasian subjects can be seen in Fig. 7.2 and this is contrasted with the different distributions found in other racial populations. For instance, in American blacks a trimodal distribution is found with a higher frequency of the Class 2 allele, and in Asian populations a decreased frequency of

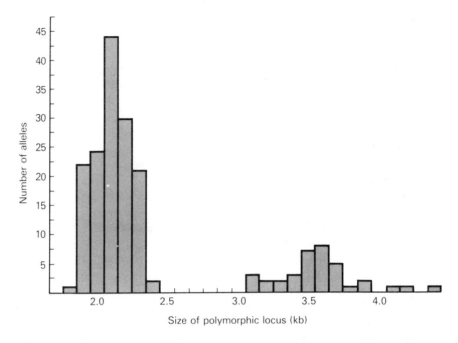

Size of polymorphic locus (kb)

Fig. 7.2 Histogram of sizes of insulin gene fragments containing class 1 and class 3 DNA insertions. (Rsa I digestion, 180 alleles).

the Class 3 allele is found compared to Caucasian subjects.

This polymorphic region is of great interest as its nucleotide sequence is unique to the human genome. Together with its proximity to the putative enhancer locus, and the non-Gaussian distribution of inserts in this region, it has been postulated that this region may be more than a genetic marker and may be a region of functional importance for the regulation of insulin gene transcription.

Only one other example has been reported of an oligonucleotide repeat region similar to the insulin gene polymorphism. It is found in the α-globin cluster between the embryonic haemoglobin genes, zeta 1 and zeta 2, and 3′ to the α-globin gene. The oligonucleotide repeat between the zeta 1 and 2 genes has been sequenced and its consensus sequence only differs by three base pairs from the insulin polymorphic repeat.

Direct evidence implicating the insulin gene polymorphism in transcription of the insulin gene is as yet lacking. Microinjection techniques using intracellular transcription systems have failed to detect any differences in insulin gene function, whether it possesses a large or short insertion of DNA. Another possibility that the region codes for a protein perhaps functioning like a prokaryote repressor or inducer is unlikely. From sequence data every third amino acid would be glycine or proline depending on which strand is transcribed.

Until there is evidence to the contrary, this polymorphism should be considered as a good genetic marker for the two parental insulin genes and as such can be used in clinical studies. The aim then is to seek for disease associations with the different insulin gene variants.

Clinical studies

Insulin gene mutants

Until 1980 only three families have been described with mutant insulins. These have all been due to amino acid substitutions within the proinsulin molecule and, therefore, due to a nucleotide substitution in the codon specifying that particular amino acid.

1. A large family was identified by Gabbay *et al.* (1976) with familial hyperproinsulinaemia and was found to be due to a mutation probably involving an arginine transversion preventing cleavage of the β chain from the C-peptide. It was inherited as an autosomal COG dominant but the affected individuals were not diabetic.

2. In 1978, a Japanese family was described where the affected individual has a mutation involving defective cleavage of the A chain from the C-peptide. The patient presented with hyperproinsulinaemia and non-insulin dependent diabetes.

3. The third mutant insulin was described by Tager *et al.* in 1979 and was due to a substitution of a leucine for phenylalanine within the β chain (at a site thought to be important for binding to the insulin receptor). The patient presented with non-insulin dependent diabetes.

Recently, two further patients have been found with β chain mutations by a novel HPLC and radioimmunoassay method. When genomic DNA was digested with the restriction enzyme MboII from the three patients with β chain mutants, variant Southern blotting patterns were observed, indicating the loss of the cutting site of this enzyme. After cloning the insulin gene alleles from one of these patients, DNA sequencing confirmed a nucleotide substitution of a cytosine to a guanine affecting the cutting sequence for MboII. This nucleotide transversion leads to the codon for phenylalanine being changed to leucine.

Disease associations found with the insulin gene polymorphic region

Type II or non-insulin dependent diabetes
    Prevalence studies. Four centres have sought for disease associations with the polymorphic region adjacent to the insulin gene, and the results

Table 7.3 Genotype distribution of the polymorphic locus adjacent to the insulin gene in Type II diabetes mellitus. Controls are significantly different from diabetics in studies (2) and (4)

| | Genotype distribution in: | | | |
| | Controls | | Type II diabetes | |
Study group	Homozygous class 1 allele $(^1/_1)$	Homozygous class 3 allele $(^3/_3)$	Homozygous class 1 allele $(^1/_1)$	Homozygous class 3 allele $(^3/_3)$
Bell *et al.* (1)	13	2	6	1
Rotwein *et al.* (2)	45	3	43	11
Owerbach and Nerup (3)	31	4	22	8
Hitman *et al.* (4)	37	7	19	20

Sources: Bell, G.I., Karam, J.H. and Rutter, W.J. (1981). *Proceedings of the National Academy of Sciences* (USA) **78**, 5758.
Rotwein, P.S., Chirgwin, J., Province, M., Knowler, W.C., Pettit, O.J., Cordell, B., Goodman, H.M. and Permutt, M.A. (1983). *New England Journal of Medicine* **308**, 65.
Owerbach, D and Nerup, J. (1982) *Diabetes* **31**, 275.
Hitman, G.A., Jowett, N.I., Williams, L.G., Humphries, S., Winter, R.M. and Galton, D.J. (1984). *Clinical Science* **66**, 383.

are summarized in Table 7.3. The most common genotype found in Caucasian populations is heterozygotes for the Class 1 and 3 alleles (1/3), accounting for 50 per cent of subjects studied; 42 per cent of subjects had the genotype homozygous for the Class 1 allele (1/1); and the rarest genotype was homozygous for the Class 3 allele (3/3), being present in less than 10 per cent of the population. Another approach is to examine the frequencies for the Class 1 and 3 alleles based on the Hardy-Weinberg principle. If the frequency of the Class 1 allele is p; and the frequency of Class 3 allele is q (and p + q = 1), then the geneotype frequencies can be calculated from the allele frequencies by the formula:

$$p^2 : 2pq : q^2$$

This assumes random mating conditions, Mendelian inheritance, and no disturbing conditions of mutation, selection or migration. The frequencies of the Class 1 allele was approximately 0.67 and Class 3 allele 0.33 in control populations from London, St. Louis, San Francisco and Copenhagen. In Type II diabetics a greater preponderance of the genotype homozygous for the Class 3 allele has been reported by some groups with an increased relative incidence of about five. An even greater preponderance of the homozygous Class 3 genotype has been found in a subgroup of diabetics who have coexisting hypertriglyceridaemia (relative incidence of 10.5).

Pedigree analysis. An alternative approach to looking for disease associations is to examine for linkage of the polymorphic inserts with diabetes in large pedigrees. In a large pedigree of maturity-onset diabetes of the young, 17 diabetics and 38 non-diabetics, Owerbach (1983) found no close linkage between DNA inserts flanking the insulin gene and

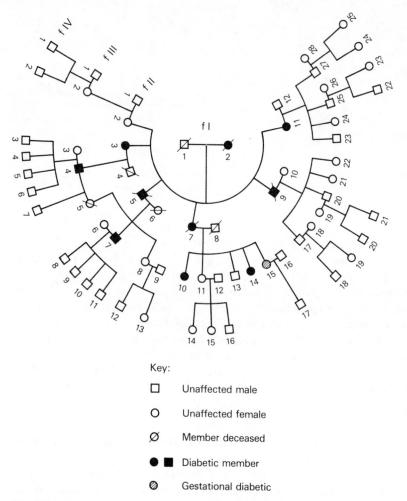

Key:

☐   Unaffected male

○   Unaffected female

∅   Member deceased

● ■ Diabetic member

⊘   Gestational diabetic

Fig. 7.3 Analysis of a large pedigree for linkage of diabetes with the polymorphic locus close to the insulin gene. The family members were genotyped using the hypervariable locus adjacent to the insulin gene and analyzed for linkage by Lod scores with an age correction and assuming an autosomal dominant mode of inheritance. Results of analysis excluded any close linkage between genotype and disease (Lod scores were -5.72 and -1.125 for recombination fractions of 0 and 0.1 respectively).

diabetes. Smaller MODY pedigrees have also been studied with no apparent association being found although they were too small to be statistically analysed. Additionally our laboratory studied a large family (11 diabetics and 56 non-diabetics) more typical of Type II rather than MODY (because of later age of onset of diabetes, 30 ± 10 years, and the presence of diabetic complications). Again no close linkage was found of the DNA inserts in the 5'-flanking region of the insulin gene with diabetes (Fig. 7.3). In conclusion, in the pedigrees so far analysed, confirmation of genetic linkage of any DNA insert near the insulin gene with Type II diabetes has not been found.

There are, however, problems with pedigree analysis in Type II diabetes. Firstly, the age of onset of the disease is very variable, being more common in the 4th and 5th decades. As one cannot confidently predict who might become diabetic this makes statistical analysis difficult when younger members are included. Secondly, as diabetic complications lead to premature death (from myocardial infarction, renal failure), key older members of the family are sometimes not available for genotyping.

Type I or insulin-dependent diabetes
Three centres have studied a total of 169 insulin-dependent diabetics with the insulin gene probe searching for disease associations with the polymorphic locus. In the largest Caucasian study from San Francisco, (Bell, 1984) Type I diabetics were compared to 83 controls. The genotype frequencies in Type I diabetics showed a greater preponderance of the homozygous Class 1 insertions (76 per cent) compared to controls of 44 per cent. Other studies have confirmed these results and are summarized in Table 7.4. The strength of the association of Type I diabetics with the genotype 1/1 is stronger than that of Type II diabetics with the genotype 3/3. Results for the linkage in Type I pedigrees are still awaited.

Table 7.4 Genotype distribution of the polymorphic locus adjacent to the human insulin gene in Type I diabetes. Genotype distributions between diabetics and controls are highly significant when tested by chi-square

	Genotype distribution in:		
Study group	Homozygous class 1 allele ($^1/_1$)	Heterozygous ($^1/_3$)	Homozygous class 3 allele ($^3/_3$)
Controls n = 88	37 (42%)	44 (50%)	7 (8%)
* Type I diabetes n = 53	42 (79%)	11 (21%)	0 (0%)
** Type I diabetes n = 113	86 (76%)	27 (24%)	0 (0%)

Source: * Hitman, G.A., Tarn, A.C. Williams, L.G. *et al.* (1984), Diabetologia **27**, 288.
         ** Bell, G.I., Horita, S., Karam, J.H. (1984). *Diabetes*, **33**, 176.

Significance of genotype distributions

The particular distribution of genotypes in populations found for this polymorphic locus adjacent to the insulin gene could have arisen by random genetic drift and the associations found with the various disease states be entirely spurious. However, there are several facts against this interpretation:

1. The non-random distribution of DNA insertional elements into two (or three) defined classes (Fig. 7.2) suggest that selective forces may be operating and that intermediate-sized insertions are in some way disadvantageous.

2. The homozygous large insertional class (3/3) is present at low frequencies in the population and shows a clear disease association with glucose and triglyceride intolerance; but

3. the same does not apply for the homozygous short insertions (1/1) which are present at a frequency of greater than 40 per cent in the healthy population and yet also show an association with a disease known to affect fertility and fecundity (Type I diabetes mellitus).

It is impossible, however, from the presently available data to account for the stage of evolution of these different genotypes. If one considers the past evolutionary history of these genotypes, the homozygous short (1/1) class may be in balance with the other genotypes, or be gradually increasing or decreasing in frequency. If the homozygous short genotype were increasing it would be very difficult to interpret its association with Type I diabetes; unless there were a subgroup of individuals with the homozygous short genotype who have an additional mutation in linkage disequilibrium that confers susceptibility to Type I diabetes. These ideas are presented schematically in Figure 7.4 showing how a beneficial

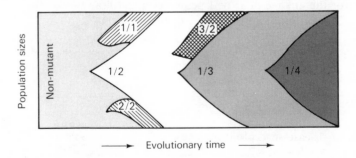

Fig. 7.4 This diagram illustrates the spread of beneficial genotypes and elimination of disadvantageous genotypes in population groups. 1/1, 1/2, 1/3, 1/4 and 2/2 are hypothetical insulin genotypes with various selective values. New mutations arise (e.g. 4), which displace other gene variants (2 and 3).

genotype may spread through a population whereas a disadvantageous one may be in the process of selective elimination. We have no way of knowing at what point in evolutionary time the present studies have been made.

Assuming that natural selection is operating on this polymorphic locus, there are several interesting possibilities.

1. The polymorphic locus is so close to the regulatory sequences on the 5'-flanking region of the insulin gene that some sized insertions may affect insulin gene transcription, leading to inappropriate rates of insulin synthesis. No differences to support this have so far been found in the first phase of insulin secretion between patients with genotype 1/1 as compared to 1/3 + 3/3.

Alternatively, the highly variable region of DNA may be acting as a genetic marker for an abnormality within the coding region for insulin producing a mutant insulin. This would be analogous to the HpaI polymorphism 3' to the β-globin gene that associates with the sickle cell mutation. Such a mutant insulin has not so far been found.

2. Some classes of DNA insertions at the polymorphic locus may be in linkage disequilibrium with other disease specific genes on the short arm of chromosome 11. A model for this interpretation would be the studies associating Type I diabetes with HLA-related antigens on chromosome 6. Initially an association with the HLA antigens B8 and B15 were found, but stronger associations have been subsequently found with HLA-DR3 and -DR4, respectively. In a similar manner the polymorphic locus on chromosome 11 may be associated with other alleles that determine susceptibility to diabetes, as yet unidentified.

3. The variable disease associations found with this polymorphic locus may be a manifestation of a polygenic disease; where other genes are required to interact before predisposition to diabetes become apparent. This is very likely to be the case with diabetes where it is known that heterogeneity exists within both Types I and II. Within each subset two or more disease susceptibility genes may be required for interaction with environmental factors before manifestation of the disease.

Future prospects

Identification of disease susceptibility genes

If the insulin gene polymorphism is in linkage disequilibrium with as yet unidentified genes that may confer predisposition can they be located by recombinant DNA techniques? By a method known as 'walking' the gene (Fig. 8.1, p. 117) it may be possible to serially select over-distant sequences from the polymorphic locus to see if they show even stronger disease associations with diabetes mellitus. If a polymorphic locus could be found that shows a one-to-one correspondence with diabetes, then this may be a possible disease susceptibility locus and could be further defined by nucleotide sequencing. Such an approach has already been used to attempt location of the gene for Duchenne muscular dystrophy on the X chromosome. A non-specific X-linked probe was initially found to have a weak linkage with the 'Duchenne gene', being about 10 centimorgans from the probe. By exploring sequences on either side of the X-linked probe further sequences have been found that are within 5 centimorgans of the possible disease gene; and it may be possible to define it further by this method (p. 116).

Use of gene probes for other aetiological factors in diabetes

Type II diabetes is considered to be a disease predominantly relating to insulin resistance and it has been postulated that abnormalities of the insulin receptor or post-receptor defects may be involved. Several groups are currently trying to clone and sequence the gene for the receptor protein for insulin in order to investigate for possible inherited defects at this site.

As more gene probes become available it may be possible to use them to identify other potential diabetogenic loci. This may enable a complete picture of the inherited components of diabetes mellitus to be obtained.

The final possibilities of gene therapy are considered in the next chapter.

Further reading

Belfiore, F., Galton, D.J. and Reaven, G.M. (1984). *Diabetes Mellitus: Etiopathogenesis and Metabolic Aspects.* Karger, Basel.
   (A collection of papers on aetiology, insulin secretion, complications and current topics in diabetes research.)
Crepaldi, G., Lefebvre, P.J. and Galton, D.J. (1983). *Diabetes, Obesity and Hyperlipidaemias.* Academic Press, London.
   (A collection of papers on the hyperlipidaemias, adipose tissue, insulin receptors and metabolic control of diabetes.)
Gabbay, K.H., De Luca, K., Fisher, J.N. *et al.* (1976). Familial Hyperproinsulinaemia: An Autosomal Dominant Defect. *New England Journal of Medicine* **294**, 911.
Tager, H., Given, B., Baldwin, D. *et al.* (1979). Structurally Abnormal Insulin Causing Human Diabetes. *Nature* **281**, 122.

8
Future developments

Discoveries in medical science unfortunately do not always go in parallel with improved health for the individual. Undoubted progress, such as vaccine therapy to eliminate smallpox or poliomyelitis from populations, or antibiotic therapy for the treatment of bacterial infections, expose the individual subsequently to a different set of diseases such as the cancers or the degenerative disorders. Drug therapy is clearly of mixed benefit. The undisputed value of such drugs as analgesics or diuretics must be offset against the many drug-induced diseases (particularly disasters like thalidomide) and the great increase in drug abuse or addiction that has occurred as a result of drug proliferation. Gene therapy arouses even more controversy, although some genetic practices have already been adopted. By genetic counselling parents are educated and advised on the nature and risks of transmitting a disease running in their family to their children, and given some estimate of the liklihood of bearing affected children. Antenatal diagnosis can be made from studies of amniotic fluid cells or foetal trophoblast to see if the foetus is affected by a severe or crippling disease, such as Down's syndrome or sickle cell disease, with the offer of an early abortion to the mother. Postnatal screening for diseases such as phenylketonuria identifies babies that require modification of their diet (a reduction of dietary phenylalanine) in order to maintain normal growth and development.

With the new information on gene structure and function, what new benefits for diagnosis or therapy may be expected for clinical practice? Genomic probes may be expected to provide more precise means for the identification of deleterious genes both in antenatal diagnosis and in postnatal screening programmes. It may even provide means to identify mutant genes for diseases in which the defective gene product is still not understood.

Diagnosis of monogenic disease
where the locus is unknown

An example of this approach is provided by Duchenne muscular dystrophy (DMD), a disorder of muscle wasting occurring in frequency of up to one in 5000 of newborn males. Although the primary biochemical defect and site of the abnormal gene locus is unknown, the disease is linked to the X-chromosome. If a DNA sequence of the X chromosome could be found that were to be closely linked to manifestations of the disease, it would be of considerable importance in the prediction of Duchenne muscular dystrophy, as well as a step towards identifying the basic biochemical defect once the presumed mutant gene had been identified. In fact, an X-chromosome sequence, defined by a restriction enzyme polymorphism, has been found that is loosely linked to the Duchenne locus (assuming that the disease is due to a single gene defect). The polymorphism occurs in 29 per cent of women in a control population and in 22 per cent of carriers for Duchenne muscular dystrophy. Although the probe sequence is not sufficiently close to the Duchenne locus to be of diagnostic value, further unique sequences may be found on either side by searching other clones with this probe that may occur closer to the abnormal locus (i.e. 'walking' the gene, Fig. 8.1).

The approach of finding a restriction fragment length polymorphism linked to a phenotypic disorder caused by a single gene defect where the primary biochemical defect is unknown, has also been applied to Huntington's chorea. This is a progressive neurodegenerative disorder with autosomal dominant inheritance. The first symptoms usually occur in the third to fifth decade with a progressive motor defect (typically chorea) and intellectual deterioration. The primary biochemical defect has never been detected. However, a DNA sequence from chromosome 4 has been found that contains two different restriction length polymorphisms; and this polymorphic DNA sequence shows close genetic linkage to the Huntington's disease locus (Lod scores >3). This DNA sequence when used as a probe may then identify the inherited locus for Huntington's chorea and eventually solve the nature of the basic gene defect. It may also have implications for patient care if the disease is clinically homogeneous and the probe can be used as a marker in other families. It will then allow accurate genetic counselling in families where Huntington's chorea segregates and where family members wish to have children. If they go on to have children it may allow antenatal diagnosis.

Both examples, Duchenne muscular dystrophy and Huntington's chorea, demonstrate the power of using linkage to DNA polymorphisms

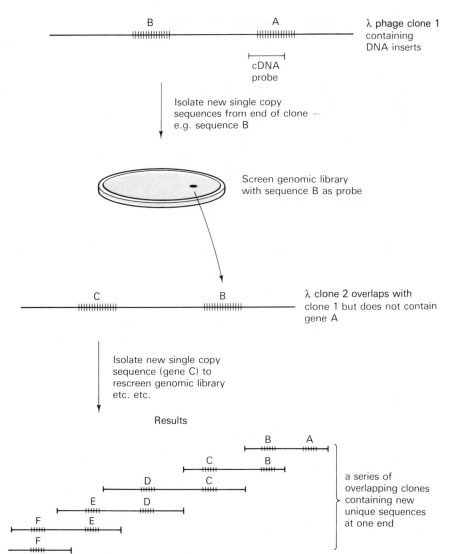

Fig. 8.1 This diagram illustrates the method of 'walking' the gene.

to study genetic diseases for which other lines of investigation have proved unsuccessful. In the future many abnormal genes from patients with metabolic diseases will become available. It is to be expected that efficient *in vitro* transcription systems will be developed to define abnormal products from these genes which may perhaps lead to better understanding of the nature of these diseases and hopefully to better lines of therapy.

Therapy involving recombinant DNA: synthesis of human insulin

A clearly established therapeutic benefit of recombinant DNA techniques is the manufacture of clinically useful gene products by genetic engineering. Insulin, for replacement therapy in insulin-dependent diabetics, has previously been obtained from the pancreas of farm animals; but can now be synthesized by fermentation processes in bacteria which contain an expression vector carrying a cloned human insulin gene. The synthesis of human insulin in bacteria starts with the isolation of cDNAs coding for the A- and B-chains of insulin respectively. In order to facilitate their insertion, and excision from a plasmid, specific restriction sites are added to each end of the synthetic gene. Substantial quantities of each chain of insulin are then generated by cloning them in *E. coli*.

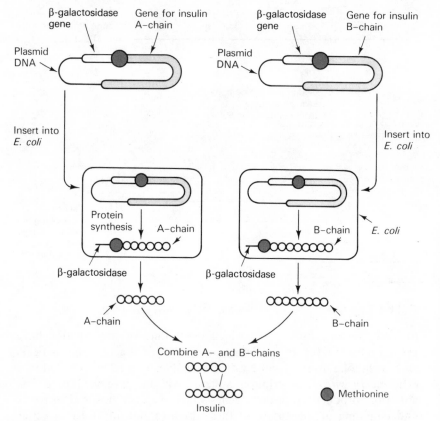

Fig. 8.2 A flow diagram for the synthesis of human insulin in bacteria (*E. coli*).

The synthetic genes for the A- and B-chains are then inserted into expression vectors to lie adjacent to a bacterial gene coding for the enzyme β-galactosidase which has been previously cloned in a plasmid. The bacteria containing the genetically engineered plasmid are cultured in large quantities and allow synthesis of the fused protein (β-galactosidase plus A- (or B-) chain of insulin). After fermentation the intact chains of insulin are liberated from the fused gene product after this has been isolated from the bacterial cells. Purification and combination of the insulin chains are required subsequently to produce functional insulin (Fig. 8.2).

The use of the β-galactosidase gene as a 'carrier' brings the production of insulin under the control of the bacterial machinery which regulates the synthesis of β-galactosidase. By growing the bacteria in a glucose-free medium containing galactose, synthesis of β-galactosidase plus insulin chains are induced, and yields are therefore increased.

An alternative approach is to assemble the DNA sequence coding for the entire human proinsulin molecule and clone it in a plasmid in a similar way to that in which the A- and B-chains are produced. Human proinsulin is then isolated, purified and the C-peptide removed by enzymic cleavage to form human insulin.

These new methods open up not only alternative means of production of insulin than from animal sources, but also increase our possibilities of investigating the physiological role of human proinsulin. Other useful protein products that could be manufactured by such engineering techniques are listed in Table 8.1

Table 8.1 Potentially useful protein products for manufacture by genetic engineering

Therapeutic category	Protein involved	Indications
Hormones	Insulin	Type I diabetes mellitis
	Growth hormone	Dwarfism
	Somatostatin	Research purposes
Anti-viral agents	Interferons	Virus infections
		? cancer
	Surface-coated antigens	Vaccines
Blood clotting	Factor VIII	Haemophilia A
factors	Factor IX	Haemophilia B
Thrombolytic agents	Streptokinase	Lysis of intravascular clots
	Urokinase	
	Fibrinolysin	
Gastrointestinal	Pancreatic lipase,	Steatorrhoea
enzymes	trypsin, amylase	
Cancer chemotherapy	Asparaginase	Leukaemia
Miscellaneous	β-endorphins	

The other therapeutic benefits that may be expected from the new genetics may depend on the type of inherited disease one considers. An approach that is useful for the rare mutation may not be applicable to the common genetic variants underlying the common metabolic diseases.

Uncommon metabolic diseases: rare mutations

It is unlikely that rare mutations, producing either the metabolic recessive or dominant disorders, will ever be completely eliminated from populations. There is an intrinsic mutation rate of DNA that generates new variants as fast as they are eliminated by natural selection; and with the recessive disorders, the carrier state (heterozygote) can become quite frequent (e.g. up to 1:25 for cystic fibrosis) since they are healthy individuals. However, there are two possible new techniques that may in the future alleviate some of the clinical burden of such rare deleterious mutation: gene switching and gene replacement.

Gene switching

During development of an individual many genes that are used during foetal growth are repressed (or switched off) after birth and a set of 'adult' genes are activated instead. Could it become possible to selectively reactivate a foetal gene that can substitute for the deleterious mutant gene in adult life?

A model for this has come from a recent study of a severe form of homozygous β-thalassaemia. This disease is characterized by a decreased or absent production of the β-subunit of adult haemoglobin, and the relative excess of α-globin molecules adversely affect red cell function and survival. Many different types of mutation of the β-globin gene (decreased gene transcription, errors in RNA splicing, premature termination of mRNA translations, etc.) have been identified. As a way of overcoming the effect of such mutations could activation of foetal globin genes for the production of γ-globin help to correct the imbalance between α-globin chains and non-α globin chains, by combining with the excess of α-chains to reform foetal haemoglobin F $(\alpha_2\gamma_2)$? Although γ-globin is normally produced during foetal life, expression of γ-globin genes decreases during the 30th week of gestation. At the same time, expression of β-globin genes increase leading to a perinatal switch from haemoglobin F to haemoglobin A production.

The nature of this 'switching' process is not clearly understood, but DNA in the region of the γ-globin genes is relatively undermethylated in cells where these genes are expressed compared to the methylated state in adult bone marrow cells where they are not expressed. This pattern of methylation has been observed for other regulated genes. 5-Azacytidine is a cytidine analogue that is incorporated into newly synthesized DNA and leads to a decrease in the activity of DNA methyltransferase reducing the methylation of newly synthesized DNA. Possibly because of its effect on the methylation of DNA, 5-azacytidine is capable of inducing cellular differentiation and can activate repressed genes in tissue culture cells. When 5-azacytidine is administered to adult animals, such as baboons, there is a transient but striking increase in foetal haemoglobin production. The drug has been administered to a patient with severe β-thalassaemia for seven days and the γ-globin synthesis increased by seven-fold, temporarily improving the patient's imbalanced globin synthesis. Erythropoiesis became more effective leading to an increase in reticulocyte count and in haemoglobin concentration. Reduced methylation of bone marrow DNA near the γ-globin genes was directly demonstrated. Of course this represents very preliminary work. The drug may have carcinogenic or other toxic effects, or it may indiscriminately activate other foetal genes, or even oncogenes; but it does raise the possibility of finding specific gene regulatory signals that may selectively activate foetal genes or genes in adult tissues that are normally repressed, to synthesize a substitute product such as an enzyme or hormone. For example, in insulin-dependent diabetics, may it be of benefit to reactivate the insulin gene, say in circulating leucocytes, to provide a continuous background secretion of insulin for the patient? Such insulin release would not of course be under control by circulating levels of blood glucose as in the β-cell of the pancreas, but still may be of use to provide a basal secretion and stabilize blood glucose levels during the 24-hour period. Other genes that may be of use to activate in tissues in which they are normally suppressed or only partially expressed in adult life are the LDL-receptor gene in common forms of hypercholesterol-aemia; or the insulin receptor gene in non-insulin dependent diabetes. These procedures may help to lower circulating levels of the abnormal metabolite (cholesterol or glucose).

Gene replacement therapy
Here the aim is more ambitious, and correspondingly more difficult, namely to replace the deleterious mutant gene by a normal one, either at the embryonic stage or in adult life. For this to work the functional human gene with its regulatory sequences must be isolated and cloned. It must be inserted into the host cell under conditions where it can function properly in the correct tissues. It may be necessary to insert it at an exact site on the host chromosome to come under the influence of the usual regulatory signals. The transformation of the recipient somatic cell must be stable and not subject to further mutations. Alternatively, it may be

possible to integrate the gene and its control sequences into a synthetic minichromosomal element and then insert it into a cell where it remains free in the cytosol as a self-replicating unit. In either situation, the transplanted gene may not be transcribed efficiently, or become unstable and undergo a cycle of mutations. The timing of gene replacement may be varied from embryo to adult. It is now possible to perform microinjection of genes into fertilized eggs (of rabbit or mouse) where the new genes are often inserted randomly in a number of linked copies. They would be expected to remain inactive unless integrated close to the normal control sequences for that gene. Such new genes have been transmitted in a normal way through at least three generations of animals. These experiments have so far all been carried out on mouse or rabbit embryos for research purposes only, although it would be possible, but quite unethical at the present stage of knowledge, to apply similar techniques to the human embryo.

Attempts have already been made to transplant human genes into adults. The prototype disease was again thalassaemia where attempts were made to transplant a normal human β-globin gene into two patients with severe β-thalassaemia. The procedure involved isolation of the normal human β-globin gene; insertion of the gene into marrow cells in tissue culture from the patient where it integrated in a random fashion with the host genome; partial irradiation of the patient's marrow to destroy defective marrow cells; and then infusion back to the patient of the transformed marrow cells previously treated with the normal β-globin gene in the hope that the treated cells could replace the remaining defective marrow cells. The treatment failed and was severely criticized on a number of grounds. There was insufficient scientific evidence to suggest that genes inserted in this manner would function properly; local hospital ethical committees did not give approval for such trials since sufficient background information on the procedure was not available; and no notification was made that recombinant DNA molecules were to be used.

However, the possibility of gene replacement remains, either into an embryo where it will be transmitted to future generations, or into an adult for treatment of a serious inherited disease. Larger issues are involved here and the Council of Europe recently reflected this in a recommendation

"... for explicit recognition in the European Human Rights Convention of the right to a genetic inheritance which has not been artificially interfered with, except in accordance with certain principles which are recognized as being fully compatible with respect for human rights ...".

Further serious debate is required to define the exact role of such new procedures.

Selective procedures to improve the genetic stock of human populations and to eliminate the unfit (eugenics) has been inextricably mixed with racialist theories. In recent years such ideas led to some of the worst excesses of the last World War, being used to justify the extermination of racial minorities. Selective breeding may still survive in the current practice of artificial insemination by donor (AID), where sperm from males of 'superior fitness' are maintained in banks for use in fertilization of women in marriages where the husband is sterile. But generally it is extremely doubtful whether artificial selective breeding practices could improve on the natural processes of evolution to benefit the genetic stock of human populations, even if they were to be ethically acceptable.

Common polygenic diseases: predicting risks

The approach here appears to be quite different from the rare mutations. The inherited component of these diseases may be part of the normal genetic polymorphisms underlying human populations. There is no benefit to be expected from their eradication; and in fact they may become advantageous in the future if environmental conditions were to change. There is, therefore, no question of antenatal diagnosis for abortion of individuals with these diseases.

Use of genomic probes for this group of diseases may have its greatest value in early detection of individuals at risk and predicting the predisposition or risks of individuals to develop these disorders in adult life, so that environmental factors may be appropriately modified. There is undisputed value in screening procedures for the early diagnosis of diabetes mellitus or hyperlipidaemia. Testing for glucose in the urine is easy to perform and is worthwhile since there are sufficient numbers of affected individuals in the population; especially at particular periods, such as pregnancy. When positive cases are found there are treatments (modified diets, oral hypoglycaemic drugs, or insulin) that are of established benefit.

Justification for the screening of hyperlipidaemias is more in dispute. The tests are slightly more difficult to perform, requiring a venepuncture and autoanalyser equipment; and although there are as many affected individuals as diabetics in the UK population, treatment is less well established. However, undoubted benefits can be obtained from dietary modification and use of the oral hypolipidaemic drugs. Some doctors recommend restricted screening for these disorders in groups of individuals at risk. This would include first-degree relatives of patients with an established familial hyperlipidaemia; subjects who have premature arterial disease in coronary, carotid or peripheral circulations; individuals in whom a severe myocardial infarction or stroke at work would endanger the lives of many people, e.g. airline pilots; and life insurance subjects with a high premium. Since one of the major complications of the hyperlipidaemias (and diabetes mellitus) is premature atherosclerosis, the earlier that subjects were to be identified the more successful therapy may be to delay the onset of arterial disease.

If the genetic polymorphisms related to the common metabolic diseases were known individuals at risk could be identified from birth. Currently the procedures for analysis of genetic polymorphism are too complex to form the basis of a screening programme; so clearly defined clinical groups would need primary consideration. These would include such ones as mentioned previously (first-degree relatives of affected subjects). As well as leading to a better understanding of the genetic determinants of these common metabolic diseases, the screening procedure would allow detection of predisposed individuals from birth onwards. Thereafter treatment would consist of modification of environmental factors to delay onset of the disease or reduce the severity of its expression. If, for example, the genotype predisposed to dietary intolerance of carbohydrate, triglyceride or cholersterol, appropriate dietary advice could be given. This would be analogous to the treatment of individuals with phenylketonuria after postnatal screening. Dietary phenylalanine is limited for the first decade of life to allow normal mental and physical development of the child. Further knowledge of the genetic determinants of the common metabolic diseases may lead to a better pharmacological approach, especially if it permits identification of new gene products that are implicated in the disease process. For example, treatment of polygenic forms of hypercholesterolaemia may benefit from therapeutic agents that induce LDL-receptor formation on cell surfaces for the removal of circulating LDL; non-insulin dependent diabetics may benefit from the induction of insulin receptors in peripheral tissues.

Thus the study of the genetic component of these common metabolic diseases may lead to delay in their onset or even prevention by modification of environmental factors. It is probable that the most important social and medical applications of genetic research in this area may lie in a better appreciation and control of the environmental factors that interact with high risk genes to produce metabolic disease.

Further reading

Burnet, M. (1971). *Genes, Dreams and Realities*. MTP Co. Ltd., Buckinghamshire.

Ley, T.J., de Simone, J., Anagnou, N.P., Keller, G.H., Humphries, R.K., Turner, P.H., Young, N.S., Heller. P. and Nienhuis, W. (1982). 5' Azacytidine Selectively Increases Gamma Globin Synthesis in a Patient with Beta+ Thalassaemia. *New England Journal of Medicine* **307**, 1469.
Weatherall, D.J. (1982). *The New Genetics and Clinical Practice.* Nuffield Provincial Hospital Trust, London.
Williamson, R. (1982). Gene Therapy. *Nature* **298**, 416.

Glossary

Abundance of a messenger RNA (mRNA) is the average number of molecules per cell usually expressed as per cent of total.

Allele is one of several alternate forms of a gene occupying a given locus on the chromosome.

Allelic variants different alleles of the same gene that may only differ from each other by one or a few nucleotides.

Alu family is a set of related DNA sequences each about 300 base pairs (bp) long dispersed throughout the human genome.

Anticodon is a triplet of nucleotides in a constant position in the structure of transfer RNA (tRNA) that is complementary to the codon(s) in mRNA to which the tRNA binds.

Apolipoproteins are a family of related proteins found as surface components on the plasma lipoproteins that assist in the transport of lipid.

Autoradiography detects radioactively labelled molecules by their effect of developing an image on an X-ray plate or photographic film.

Bacteriophage are viruses that infect bacteria; often abbreviated to phage.

Balanced polymorphism refers to the simultaneous occurrence in populations of genomes showing allelic variations (seen as either different phenotypes or changes in DNA sequences affecting the restriction pattern) that persist in constant proportions from one generation to the next.

Base pairs (bp) is a partnership of nucleotide bases of adenine (A) with thymine (T) or of cytosine (C) with guanine (G) in a DNA double helix held together by hydrogen-bonding.

Complementary DNA (cDNA) is a single-stranded DNA molecule complementary to an RNA and synthesized from it *in vitro* by reverse transcription.

cDNA library is a collection of cDNA fragments cloned in some suitable vector (e.g. plasmids of *E. coli*).

Centimorgans are units of recombination; being 1/100th of a Morgan and representing a recombination fraction of 0.01. It defines a constant probability of a crossover per unit length of chromosome and can be used to map genetic distances on a chromosome by frequencies of recombination. It is not necessarily proportional to physical length.

Chain termination is a sequence of DNA found at the end of the gene that acts as a signal for RNA polymerase to terminate transcription.

Chromosomal library a collection of cloned fragments together representing the DNA of an entire chromosome.

Chylomicra are large lipoportein particles rich in triglyceride carrying the products of digested dietary fat from the intestine to other tissues by way of the lymph and blood stream.

Cloning of DNA is the insertion of DNA into the plasmid of a bacterium or chromosome of a phage and subsequent replication to form many copies.

Coding region of DNA gives rise to a RNA molecule of similar sequence; or of mRNA giving rise to a peptide whose amino acid sequence is determined by the nucleotide sequence of the mRNA.

Codon is a triplet of nucleotides that represents an amino acid; or a termination or initiation signal.

Consensus sequence is an idealized sequence in which each position is filled by the base most often found when many actual sequences are compared.

Cosmid vectors are plasmids into which phage lambda cos sites have been inserted; as a result the plasmid DNA can be packaged *in vitro* into the phage head.

Degeneracy in the genetic code refers to the lack of effect of changing the third base of many codons on the amino acid that is represented.

Deletion mutations constitute the removal of a sequence of DNA, the regions of either side being joined together.

Disease specific genes are genes that are directly implicated in the aetiology of a disease.

DNA is deoxyribonucleic acid; a long polymer of linked nucleotides having deoxyribose as their sugar. They can form double-stranded (or helical) structures and are the fundamental substance of which genes are composed.

DNA polymorphisms are the occurrence of two or more alleles at a given chromosomal locus that may differ by one or several nucleotides. At least two of the alleles appear with frequencies greater than one per cent.

DNA primer is a short sequence of DNA (or can be RNA) that pairs with one strand of DNA and provides a free 3′-OH group at which DNA polymerase starts synthesis of a new DNA chain.

Dominant inheritance is provided by an allele that manifests its phenotypic effect in the heterozygous state.

Double helix is a possible secondary structure for DNA first proposed by Watson and Crick with two interlocking helices formed by hydrogen bonds between base pairs.

Enhancer element is a DNA sequence that facilitates the use of some eukaryotic promoters in the *cis* configuration. It can function in any location, upstream or downstream, relative to the promoter.

Eugenics a program of decreasing the frequency of harmful genes in a human population, or of increasing the frequency of advantageous genes by artificial breeding practices.

Eukaryote is an organism whose cells contain a nucleus.

Expression vector is any plasmid or phage in which foreign DNA has been inserted close to a promoter and will consequently be transcribed and translated into a protein product.

Exon is any segment of an interrupted gene that is represented in the mature RNA product.

'Fitness' of a given genotype in a given environment is measured by its relative contribution to the ancestry of future generations. It depends on both fertility and survival.

'Founder' effect is the drift effect on gene frequencies that result when a new population is founded by a small group of individuals selected from an older population.

Frequency dependent selection is selection that involves fitness differences whose intensity changes with alteration in the relative frequency of genotypes in the population.

Fused gene product; two segments of DNA derived from different genes are artificially joined together; and if transcribed and translated produce a fused product.

Gene is a segment of DNA that is involved in producing an RNA chain and sometimes a polypeptide. It includes regions preceding and following the coding region (leader and trailer sequences), as well as intervening sequences (or introns) between coding segments (or exons).

Gene banks are random collections of DNA fragments derived from the genome and carried in a suitable cloning vector.

Gene clusters are two or more genes, often derived from a common ancestral gene, located closely together in a chromosome.

Gene duplication is more than one copy on a gene of a particular chromosome.

Gene flow is the spread of genes from one breeding population to another by migration that may result in changes of gene frequency.

Gene frequencies are the proportions of a given allele out of all the possible alleles at a given locus as found in individuals of a specified population.

Gene locus is the position on a chromosome at which the gene for a particular trait is located; the locus may be occupied by any one of the alleles for the gene.

Genetic polymorphisms refers to the simultaneous occurrence in the population of genomes showing allelic variation, as seen by the production of different phenotypes or as changes in DNA sequences affecting the restriction pattern.

Gene pool is the sum total of all the different alleles in an interbreeding population at a given time.

Gene product is either the RNA or peptide molecule that results from transcription translation of the gene.

Genetic code is the set of correspondences between nucleotide triplets in DNA and amino acids in protein.

Genetic drift is the variation in gene frequency due to chance fluctuations.

Genetic linkage is the presence of two or more loci close together on a single chromosome that leads to their inheritance together. Linkage is observed only when the loci are close together since crossing-over can lead to a random assortment of loci that are far apart on the same chromosome.

Genetic markers are mutations that may have phenotypic effects or alter the restriction pattern of DNA and can be useful for tracing the chromosome on which it is located.

Genome is the total complement of genetic material in a cell.

Genomic library is a random collection of DNA fragments obtained from the total genetic material of a cell and carried in a suitable cloning vector.

Genomic probes are defined nucleic acid segments that can be used to hybridize (and therefore identify) specific DNA clones or fragments bearing the complementary sequence.

Genotype is the genetic constitution of an individual at one or more given loci.

Germ line cells are the line of cells that produce gametes.

Heterogeneous nuclear RNA (hnRNA) comprise the transcripts of nuclear genes made by RNA polymerase II; they have a wide size distribution and low stability.

Hairpin loop describes a double-stranded region formed by base-pairing between adjacent complementary sequences in a single strand of RNA or DNA.

Haplotype is a combination of alleles from closely linked loci, usually with some functional affinity found on a single chromosome.

Hardy–Weinberg principle is a rule for predicting genotype frequencies on the basis of gene frequencies under the assumptions of random mating and the absence of natural selection. The three genotypes AA, Aa and aa are present in the frequencies of p^2, $2pq$ and q^2 respectively where p and q are the frequencies of alleles A and a.

Helix is the secondary structure in which double-stranded DNA is normally organized. It consists of two interlocking helical strands held together by hydrogen-bonding between the base pairs of separate strands.

Heterozygous advantage is where a gene pair having different alleles on the two chromosomes of the diploid individual has selective advantage over individuals possessing identical alleles at this locus.

Histones are basic and small molecular weight proteins which bind to DNA.

HLA system are the histocompatibility antigens found on cells. Their genes are highly polymorphic occurring at three main loci on chromosome 6.

Homology refers to structures that have similar morphology. When referring to genes it means that they share many nucleotide sequences in common.

Human-mouse cell hybrids are cell lines resulting from the fusion of human and mouse cells and are used for studying the location of genes on human chromosomes.

Hybridization analysis is the pairing of complementary RNA or DNA strands to give either DNA-DNA or DNA-RNA hybrids; and is often used to locate DNA fragments in gene libraries or after Southern blotting.

Hydrogen bonding is the formation of weak bonds involving the sharing of an electron with a hydrogen atom. They are important in the specific pairing of bases in nucleic acids.

Inducers are environmental agents that activate the transcription of genes by binding to a regulatory protein.

Induction is the synthesis of a protein only in the presence of a specific inducer or effector molecule and involves activation of gene transcription and translation of the newly synthesized RNA into protein.

Initiation codon (AUG) is a nucleotide triplet in RNA that acts as a signal for the start of protein synthesis.

Insertion mutations are identified by the presence of additional sequences of base pairs in DNA of the genome.

Intervening sequences are segments of DNA that are transcribed but are removed from the transcript by splicing together the sequences (exons) on either side of it.

Intron-exon junctions are boundary sequences that separate coding regions from intervening sequences (introns).

Introns are intervening sequences of DNA that are spliced out of the primary transcript of RNA.

In vitro **translation systems** are a mixture of ribosomes, amino acids and all the enzymes and cofactors required for protein synthesis, to which is added RNA from an experimental source to drive peptide synthesis.

Isoenzymes are related enzymes performing similar reactions but different in structure, often by the presence or absence of a charged amino acid so that they can be resolved by gel electrophoresis.

Isomorphic forms (isoforms) are peptides with identical amino acid sequences that differ in their post-translational modification with sialyl, glucosyl or other residues.

Kilobases (Kb) is one thousand nucleotides in sequence.

Libraries are a set of cloned fragments of DNA together representing a sample of the genome.

Linkage describes the tendency of genes to be inherited together as a result of their close locations on the same chromosome.

Linkage disequilibrium is the non-random association of alleles at separate loci possibly due to a common selective basis.

Lipoproteins of plasma are small particles of lipids associated with proteins and responsible for the transport of cholesterol and triglycerides amongst the tissues of the body.

Locus is the position on a chromosome at which a gene for a particular trait resides.

Lod scores come from a statistical test to assess genetic linkage; numerically they are the ratio of the logarithm of the odds for linkage versus logarithm of odds against linkage at different recombination fractions.

Low-density lipoprotein (LDL) is a small plasma particle rich in cholesterol whose major peptide component is apoprotein B.

M13 is a filamentous DNA virus used in the DNA sequencing procedure of Sanger.

Maxam and Gilbert procedure is named from the inventors of a chemical method to determine the nucleotide sequence of DNA.

Mendelian inheritance of a trait is determined by the independent segregation of gene pairs from each other during meiosis with each gamete having an equal probability of obtaining either member of the pair. Also different segregating gene pairs assort independently and give rise to a distinctive ratio of phenotypes in successive progenies.

Messenger RNA (mRNA) is an RNA molecule transcribed from the DNA of a gene and from which a protein is translated by the action of ribosomes.

Multigenes are a family of genes with related functions located closely together on a chromosome.

Mutation describes any change in the nucleotide sequence of genomic DNA.

Nascent polypeptide chain is a newly synthesized amino acid chain attached to polysomes before post-translational modification has occurred.

Natural selection is a process favouring the reproduction of individuals that are better adapted to their environment, and tending to eliminate those unfitted.

Neutral polymorphisms are inherited variations of DNA sequences on which it is assumed that natural selection is not affecting their transmission to future generations.

'Nick translation' describes the ability of *E. coli* DNA polymerase I to use a nick in a DNA chain as a starting point from which one strand of a duplex DNA can be degraded and replaced by resynthesis with new nucleotides. It is used to introduce radioactive nucleotides into DNA *in vitro*.

Nitrocellulose filter is a paper strip made of nitrocellulose to which single stranded DNA binds firmly; used in Southern blotting and screening gene libraries.

Northern blotting is a technique for transferring RNA from an agarose gel to a nitrocellulose filter on which it can be hybridized to a complementary DNA to establish its location and size.

Nucleoside is the portion of DNA (or RNA) composed of a deoxyribose (or ribose) sugar combined with a purine or pyrimidine base.

Nucleosome is the basic subunit of chromatin consisting of about 200 base pairs of DNA and an octamer of histone protein.

Nucleotide is the portion of DNA (or RNA) composed of a deoxyribose (or ribose) sugar combined with a phosphate group and a purine or pyrimidine base.

Oligonucleotide is a linear sequence of up to about twenty nucleotides.

Operator is the site on DNA at which a repressor protein binds to prevent transcription from initiating at the adjacent promoter.

Palindromes describes a DNA sequence that is the same when one strand is read left to right or the other strand is read right to left.

Penetrance is the proportion of individuals with a specific genotype who manifest this at the phenotype level out of those with the same genotype who do not manifest it phenotypically.

Peptide bond is a covalent amide bond formed between the amino group of one amino acid and the carboxyl group of another.

Phage is a bacterial virus, abbreviated from bacteriophage.

Phage vector is a bacterial virus in which foreign DNA has been inserted for cloning purposes.

Phenotype is the observable characteristics of an organism resulting from the interaction of its genes and the environment in which development occurs.

Plasmid is an autonomous self-replicating extrachromosomal circular piece of DNA often carrying genes for antibiotic resistance.

Poly A⁺ a messenger RNA species which has a string of adenine nucleotides at the 3'-end.

Poly A⁻ a messenger RNA species which has no string of adenine nucleotides at the 3'-end.

Poly A tail is the sequence of adenine nucleotides found at the 3'-end of a eukaryotic RNA.

Polyadenylation is the addition of a sequence of adenine nucleotides to the 3'-end of a eukaryotic RNA after its transcription.

Polygenic refers to a phenotype that has been determined by two or more genes.

Polymorphism of the genome refers to the simultaneous occurrence in the population of genomes showing allelic variation. Polymorphism of proteins refers to the simultaneous occurrence of proteins showing amino acid variation. At least two of the variants should occur at a frequency of greater than one per cent.

Polyribosome is a mRNA associated with a series of ribosomes engaged in translation.

Population disequilibrium is a non-random association of genetically determined traits in a population caused by a common selective basis.

Post-translational modification is the change in chemical structure of a newly formed polypeptide, usually by addition of glycosyl, sialyl or amide residues, prior to its secretion or use in the cell.

Primary transcript is the original unmodified RNA product corresponding to a transcription unit.

Probe is a DNA or RNA molecule radiolabelled to high specific activity used to detect the presence of complementary sequences by molecular hybridization.

Prokaryotes are organisms (bacteria) that lack nuclei.

Promotor is a region of DNA involved in the binding of RNA polymerase to initiate transcription.

Pseudogenes are inactive but stable components of the genome derived by mutation of an ancestral gene.

Purine is a type of nitrogen base; the purine bases of DNA are adenine (A) and guanine (G).

Pyrimidine is a type of nitrogen base; the pyrimidine bases of DNA are cytosine (C) and thymine (T).

Reading frames are the codon sequences that are determined by reading nucleotides in groups of three from some specific fixed starting nucleotide.

Rearrangement mutations describes the change in the sequence of genomic DNA due to large sections of nucleotides changing places.

Recessive allele is an allele whose phenotypic effect is not expressed in the heterozygous state, being obscured by the dominant allele.

Recombinant DNA molecule is a novel DNA sequence formed by the covalent combination of the non-homologous DNA molecules.

Recombination is (1) any process in a diploid cell that generate new gene or chromosomal combinations not found in that cell or its progenitors; or (2) at meiosis the process that generates a haploid product whose genotype is different from either of the two haploid genotypes that constituted the meiotic diploid.

Regulatory sequences code for an RNA or protein product whose function is to regulate the expression of other genes.

Repeated DNA are DNA sequences (such as the Alu repeat) that are present in many copies dispersed throughout the genome.

Repression is the ability of bacteria to prevent the synthesis of certain enzymes when their products are present; more generally refers to the inhibition of transcription by the binding of repressor proteins to specific sites on DNA.

Repressors are proteins that bind to operators on DNA to prevent transcription.

Restriction endonucleases are a group of enzymes commonly found in bacteria that break internal bonds of DNA at highly specific points (often at or near to short palindromic sequences).

Restriction enzymes recognize specific short sequences of (usually) unmethylated DNA and cleave the duplex.

Restriction enzyme mapping is a linear array of sites on DNA that are cleaved by various restriction enzymes.

Restriction fragment length polymorphisms (RFLPs) are inherited variations in the recognition sequence of restriction endonucleases that produce different sizes of genomic fragments on Southern blotting.

Reverse transcriptase is an RNA dependent DNA polymerase enzyme.

Ribosomal RNA (rRNA) is the structural RNA associated with ribosomes as distinct from the messenger RNA (mRNA).

Ribosomes are small cytoplasmic particles made of RNA and proteins that are the sites of protein synthesis.

RNA is a polymer of ribonucleotides similar to DNA but with ribose as the sugar and uracil present instead of thymine.

RNA polymerase is an enzyme that catalyzes the synthesis of RNA using a DNA strand as template to determine the order of ribonucleotides.

RNA splicing describes the removal of introns and joining of exons in RNA; thus introns are spliced out, whilst exons are spliced together.

S-1 nuclease mapping is the use of an enzyme (S-1 nuclease) that specifically degrades unpaired (single-stranded) sequences of DNA; so DNA that has hybridized with RNA is protected and allows identification of the ends of RNA coded by the DNA transcription unit.

Satellite DNA consists of many tandem repeats (identical or related) of a short basic repeating unit.

Shine-Dalgarno sequence is part or all of the poly-purine sequence AGGAGG located on mRNA before an AUG initiation codon, and involved in binding of mRNA to ribosomes.

Signal sequence describes the role of the amino-terminal sequence of a secreted protein in attaching the nascent polypeptide to membrane prior to secretion.

Somatic mutation is the change in nucleotide sequence of genomic DNA in a body cell other than a germ-line cell.

Southern blotting is the procedure for transfering denatured DNA from an agarose gel to a nitrocellulose filter where it can be hybridized with a complementary nucleic acid. Named after its inventor Dr. E. Southern.

Splicing is the removal of introns and joining of exons in RNA.

Sucrose density gradients are a solution of sucrose whose concentration varies in a linear manner from the top to the bottom of the tube; material, when centrifuged in such a solution, will move to different positions depending on its mass.

Tandem duplications are multiple copies of the same DNA sequence arranged in series.

TATA box (Hogness) is an observed A-T rich sequence found about 25 base pairs before the startpoint of each eukaryotic transcription unit using RNA polymerase II; it may be involved in positioning the enzyme for correct initiation.

Template is a molecular 'mould' that determines the structure or sequence of another molecule; for example the nucleotide sequence of DNA determines the nucleotide sequence of RNA during transcription.

Transcription is the synthesis of RNA on a DNA template.

Transfer RNA (tRNA) is a small RNA molecule that carries specific amino acids to the ribosome during translation.

Translation is the synthesis of protein on an mRNA template.

Transposons are DNA sequences able to replicate and insert one copy at a new location in the genome.

Triplets a linear sequence of three nucleotides.

Vector for cloning is a plasmid or phage into which foreign DNA may be inserted.

Very-low-density lipoprotein (VLDL) is a triglyceride rich lipoprotein particle found in plasma and involved in the transport of endogenous triglyceride amongst tissues.

'Walking the genome' is the procedure of serially selecting ever-distant

DNA sequences from a polymorphic locus in a comprehenisve gene library to see if these more distant loci show, for example, stronger disease associations.

'Wild type' the genotype (or phenotype) that is found in nature.

Wobble hypothesis accounts for the ability of a tRNA to recognize more than one codon by unusual pairing (not G-C or A-T) with the third base of a codon.

Zygote is produced by the fusion of two gametes; it is a fertilized egg.

Index